UVEITIS I

UVEITIS

Volume I
Differential Diagnosis

Manfred Zierhut

BUTTERWORTH HEINEMANN

BOSTON LONDON OXFORD SINGAPORE

SYDNEY TORONTO WELLINGTON

Translated from the German by Thomas E. Rice

ISBN 9070-43009-6

Europe, Africa, Asia, Australia, Oceania, South and Central America

Æolus Press Science Publishers, P.O. Box 740,
4116 ZJ Buren, The Netherlands

ISBN 7506-9589-7

USA, Canada, Mexico

Butterworth-Heinemann, 313 Washington Street,
Newton, MA 02158 USA

Typeset and printed in The Netherlands by Nauta bv, Zutphen

The most pleasant challenge in my work is deletion. Once, I recall, I rose with particular satisfaction from my work, and my wife told me I looked as if I had accomplished something really extraordinary that day. I answered with pride, 'You're right! I succeeded in deleting another whole paragraph and thereby found a more rapid transition.'

Stefan Zweig

[translated from: Die Welt von Gestern. Stockholm: Suhrkamp, 1944]

Dedicated to my wife Marina
and to my daughters Sarah and Chantal.

Table of Contents

Foreword

Most ophthalmologists do not enjoy the work involved in the care of patients with uveitis, at least not as much as they enjoy the care of patients with cataract or glaucoma or retinal detachment. This is true primarily because of the imprecision associated with the diagnosis and treatment of patients with uveitis. Ophthalmologists, in general, have chosen ophthalmology as their life's work because of the precision involved in making clear, accurate diagnoses, and especially because of the precision involved in ophthalmic microsurgery. It is naturally less satisfying for the physician to have to act, to have to treat imprecisely, with a feeling of vague discomfort and fear that his or her diagnosis and treatment is not correct. Yet that is exactly the situation in which many ophthalmologists find themselves when confronted with the patient with uveitis.

The book which Dr. Zierhut has written attempts to help the ophthalmologist organize his or her thoughts with greater precision when faced with the task of caring for a patient with uveitis. This book is concise, and it outlines the various causes of uveitis, organized by principal type and location of the inflammation. Further, it suggests a targeted approach to the appropriate laboratory studies indicated for the particular type of uveitis the patient has, emphasizing not only the well-established, commonly available studies appropriate for a given patient, but also more recent advances in diagnosis currently available at specialized centers.

Dr. Zierhut emphasizes, appropriately, that establishing the underlying diagnosis in the patient with uveitis is important, since the most proper therapy depends upon the diagnosis. A further point of emphasis is the underrecognized fact that an occult systemic disease may present as uveitis, with negative systemic investigations for as long as five years before extraocular manifestations of the underlying systemic disease become detectable. Notable examples in this regard include sarcoidosis, multiple sclerosis, systemic lupus erythematosus, and limited Wegener's granulomatosis. This fact alone emphasizes the need to reevaluate patients with chronic or recurrent uveitis periodically (at least annually) rather than to declare the diagnosis as 'idiopathic' on the basis of a single evaluation.

The simplified, schematic algorithm approach to the diagnosis and therapy of patients with uveitis outlined in this concise text fulfills a great need in our pedagogic lexicon in ophthalmology, and Dr. Zierhut is to be commended for his excellent efforts in providing this resource to us.

C. Stephen Foster, M.D., F.A.C.S.
Harvard Medical School
Massachusetts Eye and Ear Infirmary
Boston

Introduction

Uveitis poses a challenge to clinicians and researchers. The present uveitis series is divided into several volumes corresponding to the primary emphases of diagnosis, therapy, and disease mechanisms. It is self-evident that neither diagnosis nor therapy can be understood without the other. Each of the two, however, has its own logic, so that a division into two volumes is justified.

When the afflicted patient presents to the ophthalmologist, differential diagnosis should be the latter's first concern. This should then be the basis for treating as specifically as possible or varying the initial therapy if required.

The second step, i.e. the therapy itself, must necessarily be oriented according to the situation and the findings in each case. Only proper diagnostic procedures can result in a meaningful, precisely targetted therapy. Uncritical treatment of all uveitis patients with steroids, especially in the absence of an adequate therapeutic concept, may indeed have broadened our information on the ocular and non-ocular side effects of these drugs; however, many publications in recent years have shown that under certain circumstances non-steroidal immunosuppressives can offer a good, if not better alternative to long-term steroid therapy.

Only the third point, i.e. a study of the mechanisms leading to uveitis, will provide new points of departure for the diagnosis and accurate therapy of uveitis. The study of immunologic patterns in recent years has already contributed a great deal to our understanding of the individual forms of uveitis. However, inasmuch as the definitive microbiological and – above all – immunologic mechanisms unfold on the molecular level, our knowledge of the mechanisms of uveitis will continue to grow only gradually.

In presenting the results of clinical and theoretical research as concisely and accurately as possible, the present series of books aims to help the practicing physician when faced with the need for concrete decisions. The series takes the most recent literature as its point of orientation. Clinical illustrations are omitted, since many subtle details can better be described than photographed, especially in the case of opacified media; and I also believe that it is more important for speedy decision-making to present the various aspects of differential diagnosis and therapy in the form of step-by-step charts.

In conclusion, I would like to thank all the colleagues who have helped me by correcting this manuscript, in particular Elisabeth Arocker-Mettinger (Vienna), Günther Grabner (Salzburg), Friederike Schmidt (Kiel), Frieder Manthey (Bordesholm), Hartmut Kuck, Martin Rohrbach, Johannes Saal, Klaus-Peter Steuhl, and Hans-Jürgen Thiel (Tübingen), Michael Raizman (Boston), Ron Neumann (Tel Aviv), and Carlos Pavesio (London).

1. The diagnosis of uveitis

1.1 Definitions

Inasmuch as many designations have established themselves over the years for the various forms of uveitis and continue to cause confusion, the following pathologic-anatomical nomenclature, recommended by the International Uveitis Study Group (1), will be used in this book:

Iritis:	An inflammatory reaction confined to the iris, with anterior chamber involvement
Iridocyclitis:	Iritis with accompanying inflammatory reaction of the ciliary body and anterior vitreous
Intermediate uveitis:	Central here is vitreous infiltration without choroidal changes, but sometimes with mild, circumscribed anterior chamber inflammation. Vascular sheathing and vascular changes may be present, occasionally with exudative retinal detachment
Pars planitis:	Inflammatory exudation in the pars plana area; this may appear within the context of iridocyclitis or intermediate uveitis
Chorioretinitis:	Exudative choroidal changes, possibly

	with secondary changes of the retina as well; these may lead to vitreous infiltration
Retinochoroiditis:	Primary retinal inflammation which spreads secondarily to the choroid
Retinitis:	Primary retinal inflammation which can lead to vitreous and anterior chamber inflammation
Panuveitis:	A combination of chorioretinitis and massive anterior chamber pathology which leads to inflammation of the entire uvea
Endophthalmitis:	Inflammation of all intraocular tissues except the globe wall, often reserved for purulent (bacterial, fungal) inflammation
Panophthalmitis:	Inflammation of the entire globe with involvement of the orbit
Anterior uveitis:	A comprehensive designation for iritis and iridocyclitis
Posterior uveitis:	A comprehensive designation for chorioretinitis and retinochoroiditis

It is important to remember that anterior uveitis can lead to optic disc swelling and/or macular edema as a complication. This does not mean, however, that the disease has turned into posterior uveitis or even panuveitis.

A further important division concerns the chronological development of inflammation. In this sense, uveitis is classified as chronic if the signs of inflammation persist for more than 3 months.

Uveitic activity is intimately connected with cellular infiltration into the anterior chamber or the vitreous. To determine the degree of infiltration, cells are counted in a 2 mm high and 1 mm wide slit lamp beam for 15 seconds. The following divisions have proven reliable:

Cells	Degree
0-5	0
6-15	1
16-25	2
26-60	3
>60	4

Although it is usually easy to count the cells in the anterior chamber and to judge whether they are old or new (size, degree of pigmentation), this may be more difficult in the case of vitreous cells. These cells are best assessed with the binocular indirect ophthalmoscope in areas where gel liquefaction has occurred. Nussenblatt and coworkers have established the following standardization of vitreal inflammatory activity (2). Finally, one should note whether the majority of cells are behind the lens, in the anterior or posterior vitreous, or peripheral.

Cells	Description	Degree
0-1	Clear	0
2-20	Slight haze	Trace
21-50	Scattered opacities	1
51-100	Pronounced opacification	2
101-250	Intensely concentrated	3
>250	Massively concentrated	4

Literature:

1. *Bloch-Michel E, Nussenblatt RB*: International uveitis study group recommendations for the evaluation of intraocular inflammatory disease. Am J Ophthalmol 103: 234-235, 1987.

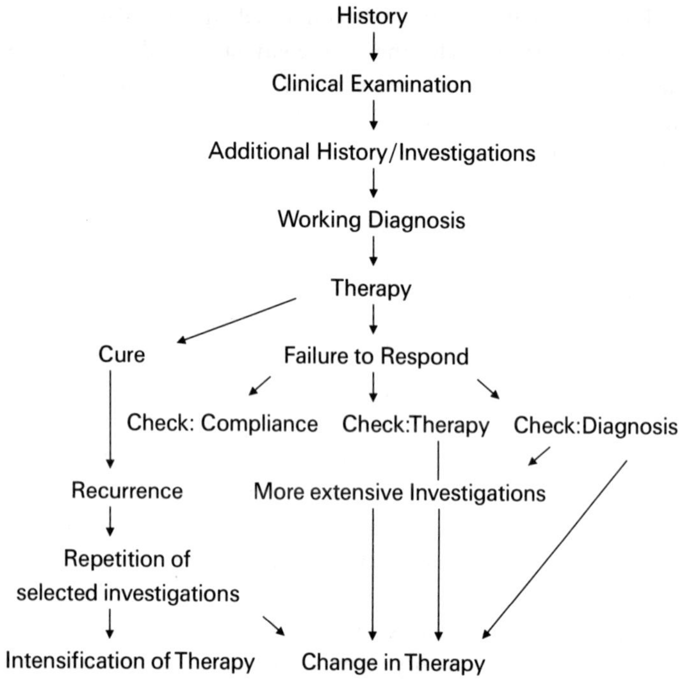

FIGURE 1: Procedure for diagnosing uveitis

2. *Nussenblatt RB, Palestine AG, Chan CC, et al*: Standardization of vitreal inflammatory activity in intermediate and posterior uveitis. Ophthalmology 92: 467–471, 1985.

1.2 Examination procedures

When a uveitis patient presents for examination, the first step after taking a clinical history is the precise evaluation of the severity of the ocular inflammation. The findings should then make it possible to classify the uveitis clinically (iritis, iridocyclitis, intermediate uveitis with or without pars plana infiltration, chorioretinitis, retinitis or panuveitis).

The next step is to query the patient anew on the history of his disease; in combination with the clinical findings, his answers should lead to a precisely targetted diagnosis. It has proven useful, especially in specialized uveitis clinics, to collect this information with the help of a standardized questionnaire. Table 1 gives an overview of possible questions, nearly all of which can be checked 'yes' or 'no'.

It is important to clarify the etiology as far as possible in order to pave the way for causal therapy (e.g. in the case of a systemic infection like syphilis) or to make prompt treatment possible in

TABLE 1: Topics for inclusion in the design of a case history questionnaire for uveitis patients

- Family history
- Social history:
  - Previous residence in a foreign country
  - Recent travel to foreign country
  - Contact with animals
  - Smoking and alcohol consumption
  - Intravenous injections or drug use
  - Bisexual or homosexual contacts
  - Profession
  - Present medication if any
- Previous history:
  - Any illnesses which can be forerunners of uveitis/retinitis/vasculitis
  - Specific symptoms: (symptoms of the head and neck, the skin, the respiratory tract, the blood, the gastrointestinal tract, the bones and joints, the GU-tract)
- Pregnancies:
  - Present or planned pregnancy
- Psychological history:
  - Stress, psychiatric care

case of a still inconspicuous, typically related illness (e.g. ankylosing spondylitis in acute HLA-B27-positive anterior uveitis). At the end of the diagnostic procedure, the etiology of the uveitis should be clear, or at least a working (suspected) diagnosis should be on hand. This working diagnosis should either take a firm shape or change as time goes on. Since intraocular inflammation can be the presenting symptom in systemic disease, it is also important to carry out repeated investigations when caring for such patients.

Example:
In the case of a patient with iridocyclitis and confirmed elevated angiotensin converting enzyme (ACE) but negative chest X-ray and gallium scan, the rest of the overall clinical picture gives no indications of sarcoidosis. In case of recurrences in such a patient, further ACE tests are recommended, together with chest X-rays and gallium scan imaging for early detection of lung or lacrimal gland involvement.

The art of diagnosing uveitis consists in casting doubt on working diagnoses until an etiology has been confirmed. As the illness develops, the patient may shift from one etiological category into another which better characterizes his uveitis.

Example:
A patient with acute anterior uveitis who is HLA-B27-positive (but without signs of systemic disease) would automatically be classified etiologically in a specific group (cf. Chapter 3.5). However, a HLA-B27-positive patient can of course also develop herpetic keratouveitis; in this case, he would belong to a different etiological group and no longer be classified among those with HLA-B27-positive anterior uveitis, provided that he develop no further illnesses associated with HLA-B27.

As a means of maintaining perspective when confronted with the often voluminous files of these patients, it is useful to start a checklist on the course of the disease for every new patient and maintain it conscientiously by pencil (for easy erasure in case of changes) (Table 2). Such a checklist gives a quick overview of the previous development of the disease, especially when the patient has not been seen for some time.

TABLE 2: 'Uveitis-file' checklist

- Working diagnosis
- Date of onset of the disease
- Number of recurrences
- Diagnosis
  - HLA
  - Lues serology
  - Most recent ACE
  - Most recent chest X-ray
  - Serology tests
- Most recent internal examination
- Other findings
- Most effective therapy to date
- Complications of the disease/therapy

The next step is to initiate a diagnostic procedure for uveitis based on the overall clinical picture and the case history. To save costs, the extent of the diagnostic procedure should also correspond to the severity of the disease. Thus, HLA-B27 typing is unnecessary in the case of a female patient with no clinical signs of HLA-B27-related illness (cf. chapter 3.1), provided that a newly discovered anterior uveitis is present which can be easily controlled with local steroids. If justified by the overall degree of discomfort, however, HLA-B27 testing is required even in the case of a first onset of illness. In view of the expense of many examination procedures, superfluous diagnostic steps or those of no particular consequence should be omitted. The more precisely cases of uveitis are etiologically classified, the sooner is it possible to make comparisons regarding therapy, pattern of development, and prognosis. The following chapters take up the most important techniques in the diagnosis of uveitis.

1.3 Diagnostic examination methods

1.3.1 Routine laboratory testing

Laboratory tests are basic to the diagnostic procedure in every first examination of a uveitis patient and should include the following:

- Blood count (differential blood count only if there is a precise indication of e.g. eosinophilia or leukemia)
- Liver enzymes
- Kidney function parameters (creatinine, urea)
- ESR
- In case of systemic therapy of uveitis, these parameters must be checked as a guide to therapy (cf. Vol. 2)

1.3.2 Antibody tests

a) Serum

Serologic antibody tests are important for the differential diagnosis of uveitis. Because of the prevalence of infectious microorganisms in the population, however, the information value of an antibody titer against some microorganisms is limited. On the other hand, negative titers do not necessarily indicate that the corresponding microorganisms can be excluded as initiators of an uveitis. A description and evaluation of serologic examinations will be included in the respective clinical picture of each case.

b) Aqueous and vitreous samples

The ratio of antibody (Ab) titers in the anterior chamber (AC) or vitreous puncture specimen in comparison with the serum-antibody titer indicates possible intraocular antibody production. In this regard, the Goldmann-Wittmer Quotient (Q) is calculated as follows:

$$Q = \frac{\text{AC-Ab}}{\text{Serum Ab}} : \frac{\text{AC-immunoglobulins}}{\text{Serum-immunoglobulins}}$$

Since the anterior chamber titer also depends on the condition of the iris vessels and their permeability, the titer of a serum constituent in the anterior chamber and the serum which is certainly not produced in the anterior chamber is also determined as an aid in measuring permeability. This is usually albumin or – as in the above formula – the total immunoglobulin level.

Evaluation: If the quotient is 1, the antibodies in the anterior chamber stem from the serum; if it is above 1, then an intraocular antibody production is to be assumed. Antibody levels found in the anterior chamber or the vitreous puncture specimen have proven to be important diagnostic criteria, especially in viral diseases of the uvea and the retina (herpes simplex, varicella zoster).

Literature:

1. *Dussaix E, Cerqueti PM, Pontet F, Bloch-Michel E:* New approaches to the detection of locally produced antiviral antibodies in the aqueous of patients with endogenous uveitis. Ophthalmologica (Basel) 194: 145-149, 1987
2. *Kaplan HJ, Lee FK, Waldrep JC, Nahmias AJ, Stulting RD:* Viral antibodies in the aqueous humor in idiopathic uveitis. In: Uveitis update. Saari KM (Ed.) Elsevier, Amsterdam, pp. 437-441, 1984

1.3.3 Autoantibodies

a) Antinuclear antibodies

Antinuclear antibodies (ANA) are found in 80-90% of patients with juvenile arthritis and uveitis. Their determination is important, since the ANA-positive type of juvenile uveitis in particular has a relatively poor prognosis and requires early, aggressive therapy (cf. Vol. 2). Antinuclear antibodies are also found in various systemic diseases, e.g. in systemic lupus erythematosus (nearly 100%), Sjögren's syndrome (97%), dermatopolymyositis (up to 40%), progressive scleroderma (90%), CREST syndrome (96%), psoriasis (30%), lung fibrosis, alveolitis (60%), immune thrombocytopenia (70%), autoimmune-hemolytic anemia (50%), chronic aggressive hepatitis (70%), primary biliary cirrhosis (40%), autoimmune thyroiditis (40%), leukemia (70%), and mononucleosis (70%).

b) Anticardiolipin antibodies

These lead to thrombosis in the anti-phospholipid syndrome and are also found in lupus erythematosus, the Guillain-Barré syndrome, Huntington's chorea, Behçet's disease, and AIDS. Determination of them should be carried out when occlusive retinal vasculitis of unclear origin is present.

c) Antineutrophilic cytoplasmic antibodies (ANCA)

ANCA can be divided into c-ANCA (classical) with a cytoplasmic pattern of fluorescence, and p-ANCA, with a perinuclear pattern of fluorescence. c-ANCA are found in 90-100% of patients with active Wegener's disease and possibly appear in Churg-Strauss syndrome and other forms of systemic vasculitis as well, although this is not yet definitively established, but interestingly, also in appr. 10-15% of uveitis patients without further signs of Wegener's disease. p-ANCA are found in Wegener's disease (5%), Churg-Strauss syndrome, lupus erythematosus, chronic polyarthritis, periarteritis nodosa, ulcerative colitis, Crohn's disease, and glomerulonephritis and recently more often in ocular and orbital Wegener's disease. Whereas a c-ANCA is practically proof of Wegener's disease, no clear significance is presently assigned to p-ANCA. The titer of c-ANCA correlates with disease activity, and can be used as a measure of therapeutic efficacy.

d) Rheumatoid factor

The test for rheumatoid factor is carried out together with that for antinuclear antibodies and HLA-B27. It is significant only for the differentiation of juvenile arthritis from anterior uveitis and is usually negative in the HLA-B27-negative, ANA-positive group. Rheumatoid arthritis (positive rheumatoid factor) practically never leads to uveitis, except in the presence of scleritis.

e) Anti-streptolysin titer

Irrelevant for the diagnosis of uveitis or its differentiation.

Literature:

1. Van der Woude FJ, Lobatto S, Permin H, et al.: Autoantibodies against neutrophils and monocytes: tool for diagnosis and marker of disease activity in Wegener's granulomatosis. Lancet 1: 425-429, 1985
2. *Glacet-Bernard A, Bayani N, Chretien P, et al:* Antiphospholipid antibodies in retinal vascular occlusions. Arch Ophthalmol 112: 790-795, 1994

1.3.4 HLA testing

The HLA system comprises numerous surface antigens required

for the activation of T cells. Some of these antigens appear more frequently in certain diseases; the pathophysiologic mechanism of this remains unclear. An important role in the diagnosis of uveitis is established for HLA-B27 in acute anterior uveitis and HLA-A29 in birdshot retinochoroidopathy and, with certain reservations, for HLA-B51 in Behçet's disease (in Japan: 57% of patients are positive, compared to 12% of controls; in Germany: 67% of patients are positive, compared to 6% of controls; in the USA: 12% of Caucasian patients with Behçet's disease are positive, compared to 10% of controls).

Other serologic associations which have been described are considerably less helpful for differential diagnosis. Associations which can be identified with the help of molecular-biologic methods are still in the experimental testing stage and are too expensive for routine use. HLA-B27-positive antigen in uveitis other than acute anterior uveitis provides no information about the case in question, since no association with other forms of uveitis has been proven to date.

Literature:

1. *Kötter I, Dürk H, Fierlbeck G et al:* Behcet's disease in 39 German and Mediterranean patients. In: Godeau P, Wechsler B (editors): Behcet's Disease. Elsevier Science Publishers Amsterdam, pp. 197-200, 1993
2. *Nussenblatt RB, Palestine AG:* Uveitis. Fundamentals and clinical practice. Year Book Medical Publishers, pp. 24-32, 1989
3. *Wakefield D, Montanaro A, McCluskey P:* Acute anterior uveitis and HLA-B27. Surv Ophthalmol 36: 223-232, 1991

1.3.5 Biopsy

a) Conjunctival biopsy

Indications:
Conjunctival biopsy is significant only in sarcoidosis, but should be carried out only in the case of visible, granulomatous changes, since 'blind' biopsy seldom leads to a positive result. The conjunctival biopsy is positive in 50% of all cases where sarcoidosis at another site has already been histologically confirmed.

Procedure:
After forming a bleb with the injected local anesthetic this bleb is dissected. At least for immunohistochemical studies one should try to touch the tissue as little as possible.

b) Lacrimal gland biopsy

Indications:
This is carried out on uveitis patients only when sarcoidosis is suspected. However, the biopsy is recommended only in case of an enlarged lacrimal gland or positive gallium enrichment and only if biopsy from other sites has not yet confirmed the diagnosis.

Procedure:
The recommended technique today is that of Weinreb et al.(3). Here one uses a transconjunctival approach for biopsy of the superficial palpebral lobe tissue.

c) Retinal and choroidal biopsy

This form of biopsy should be reserved for rare diagnostic problem cases, since it can provoke retinal detachment.

Indications:

If the fellow eye is threatened by blindness and there is no etiological indication of a promising line of therapy, or the disease remains unaffected by treatment to date (e.g. steroids, broad-spectrum antibiotics, or acyclovir).

Procedure:

External or internal biopsy.

Distribution:

The biopsy should be divided into three parts:

1. 20%: microbiological examinations, including tissue cultures as required (prior to this, precise information concerning the transport medium should be obtained from a microbiological laboratory).
2. 40%: frozen in liquid nitrogen for tissue diagnosis using monoclonal antibodies.
3. 40%: in 4% glutaraldehyde for routine light and electron microscopy.
4. Size: 4 × 2–3 mm

Biopsies in retinitis have been superseded in many cases by the PCR technique (cf. Chapter 1.3.6).

Literature:

1. *Nichols CW, Eagle RC, Yanoff M, Menocal NG:* Conjunctival biopsy as an aid in the evaluation of the patient with suspected sarcoidosis. Ophthalmology 87: 287–291, 1980
2. *Nussenblatt RB, Davis JL, Palestine AG:* Chorioretinal biopsy for diagnostic purposes in cases of intraocular inflammatory diseases. Develop Ophthalmol 23: 133–138, 1992
3. *Weinreb RN, Tessler H:* Laboratory diagnosis of ophthalmic sarcoidosis. Surv Ophthalmol 28: 653–664, 1984

1.3.6 Anterior chamber puncture

Indications:

- In case of suspected pathogens
- In testing for antibodies (cf. Chap. 1.3.2)

Procedure:

- 25-30 gauge needle (insulin syringe)
- Yields ca. 100-200 μl of fluid
- Before or after the puncture, serum must also be withdrawn for determination of antibody titers (to test for the Goldmann-Wittmer coefficient) (cf. Chap 1.3.2)

Methods of identifying pathogens:

- Culture (more than 2 cultures cannot be used; these should be selected before the puncture)
- Polymerase chain reaction (PCR)
  - DNA-fragments with a known nucleotide sequence will be detected by amplification using primers
  - high specificity and sensitivity

Literature:

1. *Fox GM, Crouse CA, Chuang EL, et al:* Detection of herpes virus DNA in vitreous and aqueous specimens by the polymerase chain reaction. Arch Ophthalmol 109: 266–271, 1991
2. *Garweg J, Fenner T, Schmitz H, Böhnke M:* Nachweis von HCMV-DNA im Kammerwasser zur Diagnosesicherung der viralen Retinitis. Fortschr Ophthalmol 88: 735–739, 1991

1.3.7 Diagnostic vitrectomy

Indications:

- In testing for antibodies (cf. Chap 1.3.2)
- For cytologic diagnosis and culture:
  - when specific pathogens are suspected (endophthalmitis, postoperative uveitis, nematodes)

- when tumors are suspected
- In case of resistance to therapy

Procedure:

- Pars plana vitrectomy:
  - advantage: observation during surgery
  - disadvantage: sample is diluted, but can be undiluted if first sample is taken in syringe without infusion

or

- Direct vitreous puncture:
  - advantage: undiluted, with a yield of 200-300 μl, especially recommended for aphakic eyes (use a 22-gauge needle)
  - disadvantage: may result in vitreo-retinal traction
- Separation into fluid and culture (antibody tests) and cells (for culture or immedate tests)
- In case of vitrectomy: use a membrane filter (0.2 μm) for enrichment

Methods of identifying pathogens:
cf. Chap 1.3.6

Literature:

1. *Engel HM, Green WR, Michels RG, et al:* Diagnostic vitrectomy. Retina 1: 121-149 1981
2. *Freeman WR, Schneiderman TE:* Invasive posterior segment diagnostic procedures in immunosuppressed patients. Int Ophthalmol Clin 29: 119-126, 1989

1.3.8 Radiological investigations

a) Chest X-ray

This is an indispensable component of any basic examination carried out in the case of doubtful uveitis to exclude the presence of tuberculosis or sarcoidosis.

b) X-ray of the sacroiliac joint

Involvement of the sacroiliac joint is found in the various forms of seronegative spondylarthritis (e.g. ankylosing spondylitis, Reiter's disease, psoriatic arthropathy, Crohn's disease, or arthritis in association with ulcerative colitis).

Indications:
Stiffness or deep-seated back pain, particularly in the early morning.

c) Gallium scan

This test is more sensitive for sarcoidosis than a lung X-ray. Gallium citrate deposits are formed above all on activated macrophages, which seem to play an important role in sarcoidosis. Gallium is found stored in the lacrimal gland in 60–75% of all sarcoidosis patients. The scan is also positive in tuberculosis, carcinomas, and lymphomas.

Indications:
Due to the relatively high radiation exposure, gallium scanning should only be carried out if sarcoidosis is suspected (e.g. in borderline or high ACE in the absence of X-ray confirmation, when there is no biopsy or when acute sarcoidosis-uveitis is clinically suspected).

Because of the radiation exposure, the indications should be weighed carefully if the patient is a child.

Literature:

1. *Karma A, Poukkula AA, Ruokonen AO:* Assessment of activity of ocular sarcoidosis by Gallium scanning. Br J Ophthalmol 71: 361–367, 1987
2. *Weinreb RN, Barth R, Kimura SJ:* Limited Gallium scans and angiotensin converting enzyme in granulomatous uveitis. Ophthalmology 87: 202–209, 1980

3. *Weinreb RN, Yavitz EQ, O'Connor GR:* Lacrimal gland uptake of Gallium Citrate GA 67. Am J Ophthalmol 92: 16–20, 1981

1.3.9 Other immunologic testing methods

a) Immunoglobulin tests

Determination of total immunoglobulins has no relevance for the diagnosis of uveitis.

b) Immune complexes

The immune complexes have no clear information value in the diagnosis of uveitis, but may be useful as parameters of the development of systemic vasculitis.

c) Complement components

An examination of individual components is worthwhile only if there is suspicion of congenital complement defects or an increased complement consumption appears likely.

C3, C4: Deficiency resulting in an increased susceptibility to bacterial diseases and immune complex-mediated diseases

CH50: Total hemolytic activity is reduced in active lupus erythematosus or acute generalized immune complex vasculitis.

d) T-cell subpopulations

Determination of T-cell subpopulations in anterior chamber or vitreous puncture specimens does not assist in diagnosis or affect the therapy. Determination in the blood is useful in case of T cell deficiency.

e) Anti-retinal-S-antigen antibodies

This test is interesting at present only in the context of scientific research, since no current consensus exists as to whether the demonstration of anti-retinal-S-antibodies is to be viewed as a negative sign (attack on retinal S-antigen) or a positive one (protection of the retinal S-antigen).

f) Eye-unspecific autoantibodies

Unspecific stimulation of autoantibodies appears to ensue in infectious processes. Among these autoantibodies, different ones are also found in anterior uveitis (with predilection for anti-sarcolemma, antimicrosomal, and anti-laminin antibodies) and in posterior uveitis (with predilection for anti-endothelial autoantibodies), but only rarely in intermediate uveitis.

Literature:

1. *Belfort RU, Moura NC, Mendes NF:* T and B lymphocytes in the aqueous humor of patients with uveitis. Arch Ophthalmol 100: 465-467, 1982
2. *Forrester JV, Stott DI, Hercus KM:* Naturally occurring antibodies to bovine and human retinal S-antigen: a comparison between uveitis patients and healthy volunteers Br J Ophthalmol 73: 155-159, 1989
3. *Murray PI, Dinning WJ, Rahi AHI:* T-Lymphocyte subpopulations in uveitis. Br J Ophthalmol 68: 746-749, 1984
4. *Zierhut M, Klein R, Berg P, Waetjen R, Frohn A, Thiel HJ:* Serum autoantibodies in uveitis. In: World Uveitis Symposium. Belfort R Jr, Petrilli AMN, Nussenblatt R (editors). Roca, Sao Paulo 159-165, 1989

1.3.10 Other serologic test parameters

a) Angiotensin converting enzyme (ACE)

This enzyme is found mainly in endothelial cells of the lung capillaries and alveolar macrophages; however, it also develops in granuloma-forming epithelioid cells. It is elevated by 60–90% in active sarcoidosis, but rarely in other lung diseases. Children may display physiologically elevated ACE values. Steroids suppress elevated ACE activity.

b) Lysozyme determination

Lysozyme is formed primarily in granulomas and is therefore found in greater amounts in the serum in granulomatous diseases such as sarcoidosis, tuberculosis and leprosy.

Literature:

1. *Baarsma GS, La Hey E, Glasius E, et al:* The predictive value of serum angiotensin converting enzyme and lysozyme levels in the diagnosis of ocular sarcoidosis. Am J Ophthalmol 104: 211–217, 1987
2. *Weinreb RN, Kimura SJ:* Uveitis associated with sarcoidosis and angiotensin converting enzyme. Am J Ophthalmol 89: 180–185, 1980
3. *Weinreb RN, Tessler H:* Laboratory diagnosis of ophthalmic sarcoidosis. Surv Ophthalmol 28: 653–664, 1984

1.3.11 Skin tests

Positive result: Shows a delayed immune reaction to the corresponding antigen (e.g. Mycobacteria).
Negative result (anergy): lack of previous exposure, sarcoidosis, herpes zoster. The reaction takes place depending on age, simultaneous steroid therapy, and the presence of neoplastic disease.

Tuberculin test: A negative result does not exclude tuberculous uveitis in all patients.
Histoplasmosis skin test: Is no longer used.
Kveim test (in diagnosis of sarcoidosis): is no longer used.
Skin test: Useful if there is suspicion of brucellosis, cryptococcosis, or coccidioidomycosis.

1.3.12 Urine analysis

Used to test elimination by the kidneys and meaningful only in the case of specific problems with kidney involvement or where vasculitis is suspected.

1.3.13 Stool examination

Indications:

- Suspicion of parasitic uveitis (Entamoeba histolytica, Giardia lamblia).
- Toxocara canis is almost never found in the stool.

1.3.14 Fluorescein angiography

Indications:

- Every recurrent intermediate and posterior uveitis noted as the initial picture; serves to identify possible complications on a comparative basis
- Assessment of the activity of vasculitic components
- The fluorescein angiographic staining pattern can constitute an important criterion in distinguishing the so-called 'white-dot syndrome' (cf. pp. 72-86)
- A help in the differential diagnosis of primary choroidal or retinal processes
- Macular edema and disc edema
- Subretinal neovascular membrane
- Indocyanine green angiography may be helpful in the differentiation of chorioretinal diseases in the future

Literature:

1. *Gass JDM:* A fluorescein angiographic study of macular dysfunction secondary to retinal vascular disease. Arch Ophthalmol 80: 606–617, 1968
2. *Listhaus AD, Freeman WR:* Fluorescein angiography in patients with posterior uveitis. Int Ophthalmol Clin 30: 297–308, 1990

1.3.15 Electrophysiological tests

Deviations from the normal electroretinogram (ERG) appear to reflect the extent of tissue destruction. ERG and EOG may be helpful in the differential diagnosis of some white-dot syndromes.

Literature:

1. *Hatt M, Niemeyer G:* Elektroretinographie bei Morbus Behçet. Graefes Arch klin exp Ophthalmol 198: 113–120, 1976
2. *Lawwill T, Wacher W, MacDonald R Jr:* The role of electroretinography in evaluating posterior uveitis. Am J Ophthalmol 74: 1086–1093, 1972

1.3.16 Immunohistochemical tests

These tests should be carried out in the case of conjunctival and scleral biopsies to exclude vasculitis if uveitis is present with scleritis or episcleritis. The tests are called for whenever a biopsy is taken from the retina or choroid. Stainings should be made for IgG, IgM, IgA, fibrinogen and complement component C3, and possibly for a determination of T-cell subpopulations and to show the presence of HLA-class II or IL-2r expression, which is evidence of an activated T cell response.

Literature:.

1. *Foster CS:* Cicatricial Pemphigoid. Trans Am Ophthalmol Soc 84: 527–663, 1986

2. *Pepose JS:* Infectious retinitis. Diagnostic modalities. Ophthalmology 93: 570–573, 1986

1.3.17 Search for foci of inflammation

The search for latent foci of inflammation is now regarded as obsolete. The patient should be examined by an otorhinolaryngologist if he complains, e.g. of frequent throat pain and tonsillectomy has been recommended because of manifest tonsil changes. The teeth should be cared for if the dentist recommends it, but this should not involve extirpation of entire rows of teeth because of uveitis, as was often the case in earlier days.

1.4 Minimal diagnostic procedure for uveitis (screening)

a) Initial manifestation of uveitis

- Chest X-ray
- Simple blood count
- ACE
- HLA-B27 in severe acute anterior uveitis
- Children: ANA, HLA-B27
- Lues serology
- then additional diagnostic procedures as specified by history and physical findings

b) Recurrent anterior uveitis

- Differential blood count
- HLA-B27
- Lyme disease
- Gallium scan when there is clinical suspicion of sarcoidosis but no previous histologic confirmation
- In some cases, anterior chamber puncture (e.g. if HSV is suggested)

- ANA
- Tuberculin test if no earlier inoculation took place
- plus all listed in a)

c) Intermediate uveitis

- Lyme disease
- Gallium scan when there is clinical suspicion of sarcoidosis but no previous histologic confirmation
- Tuberculin test if no earlier inoculation took place
- plus all listed in a) without HLA-B27

d) Posterior uveitis

- Toxoplasmosis serology if there is a retinal lesion to suggest toxoplasmosis
- Toxocara serology if toxocara is suspected
- Lyme disease
- Tuberculin test if no earlier inoculation took place
- HLA-A29 if birdshot retinopathy is suspected
- HLA-B51 if there is clinical suspicion of Behçet's disease
- Gallium scan where there is clinical suspicion of sarcoidosis but no previous histological confirmation
- Vitreous puncture in case of therapy resistance
- Retinal biopsy if the fellow eye is threatened and the first eye severely damaged
- plus all listed in a) without HLA-B27

e) Retinitis

- Serology: HIV, HSV, VZV, toxoplasmosis, further serological tests depending on the total picture
- In case of resistance to therapy: vitreous puncture
- Retinal biopsy if the fellow eye is threatened and the first eye severely damaged

f) Vasculitis

- Differential blood count
- ANA, anti-phospholipid antibodies
- Gallium scan where there is clinical suspicion of sarcoidosis but no previous histological confirmation

g) Uveitis with scleritis

- ANCA
- ANA
- Tuberculin test if no earlier inoculation took place
- Sputum test for a more specific diagnosis of tuberculosis if this is suspected clinically
- Immunohistochemical examination of a conjunctival biopsy if there is clinical suspicion of vasculitis
- Rheumatoid factor

2. Tables of differential diagnosis

The tables which follow in this chapter are intended to describe and distinguish the most significant forms of uveitis from one another. They have been designed in such a way that clinicians, for example, are guided from slit lamp or fundus findings to a tentative diagnosis which can then be differentiated or substantiated through further laboratory tests. Chapter three then goes into an assessment of the individual laboratory parameters of each clinical picture.

The aim of these tables is to make the most efficient possible use of each criterion for purposes of etiological diagnosis and thus therapy as well. In view of the multitude of causes of uveitis, it is impossible to take all possible causative factors into consideration, especially since some clinical pictures have been described in only a few patients. Although some uveitis signs are often found in some entities, these signs are almost never pathognomonic.

2.1 Anterior uveitis (Figures 2 and 3)

Whereas only about 6% of the central European population is HLA-B27-positive, this surface marker is found in approx. 40-60% of patients with acute anterior uveitis. Although it is still unclear, for the most part, why HLA-B27 leads to uveitis, and above all to anterior uveitis alone, it appears justifiable for clinical reasons to divide anterior uveitis into a HLA-B27-positive and a negative group during the course of diagnosis. Even in case of HLA-B27-positive anterior uveitis without systemic disease, such a disease could develop later and explain the uveitis.

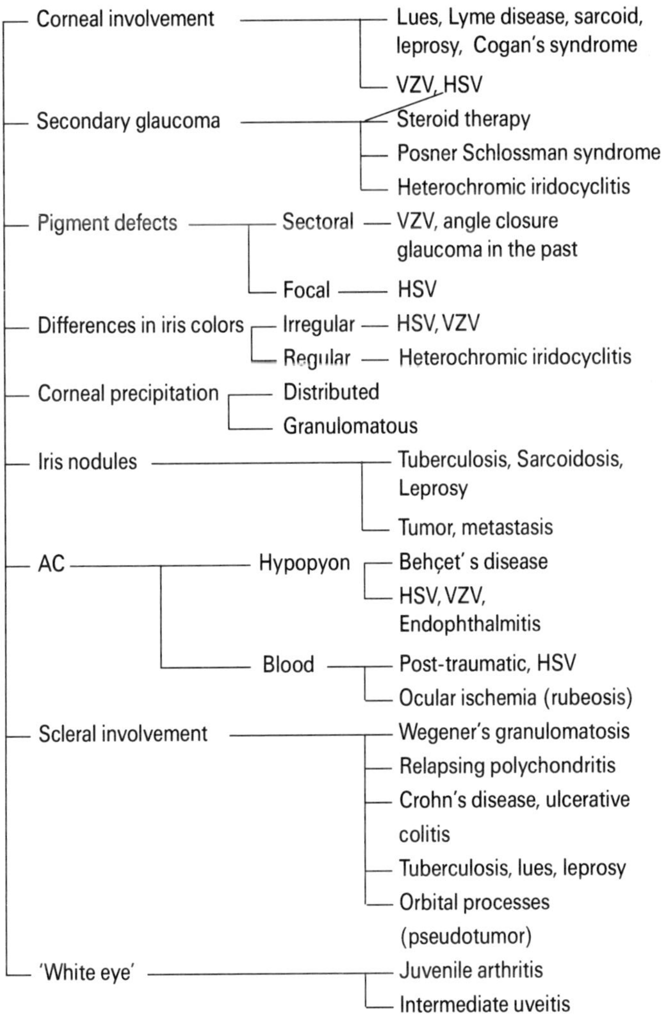

FIGURE 2: Clinical anterior uveitis

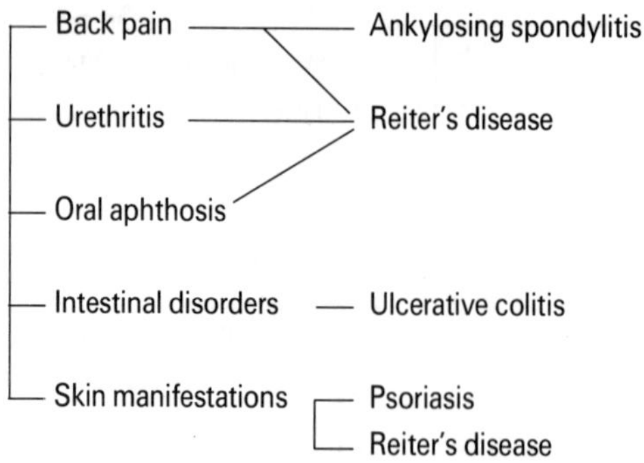

FIGURE 3: Anterior uveitis and HLA-B27

2.2 **Intermediate uveitis** (Figure 4)

The list of causes of intermediate uveitis is relatively short. Toxocara and toxoplasmosis can be taken into consideration if the view of the fundus is severely obscured. Among diseases to be considered most often are sarcoidosis and multiple sclerosis, rarely Lyme disease.

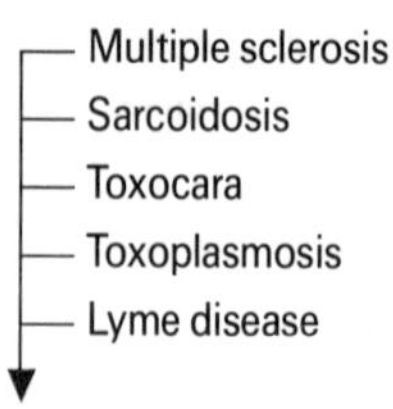

FIGURE 4: Intermediate uveitis

2.3 **Chorioretinitis** (Figure 5)

Lues, sarcoidosis, tuberculosis, Lyme disease, an atypically developing toxoplasmosis, and in children toxocara infection should be systematically eliminated as possibilities in every case of chorioretinitis. The next step is to distinguish between geographical and punctate changes. These changes are generally grouped under the term 'White-dot syndrome' (cf. Chap. 2.4). If cxudativc dctachmcnt is found in conjunction with chorioretinitis, this is most likely an indication of Vogt-Koyanagi-Harada syndrome. Chronic progression in the elderly is suggestive of intraocular lymphoma.

- Sarcoidosis, lues, TB, Lyme disease, toxoplasmosis, toxocara
- Geographical changes — Serpiginous chorioiditis
  - Good visual acuity-APMPPE
  - Vogt-Koyanagi-Harada syndrome, sympathetic ophthalmia
- Exudative detachment (→ Vogt-Koyanagi-Harada syndrome)
- Punctate changes — White-dot syndromes (see figure 6)
- Vitreous or ant. chamber cells — Multifocal chorioretinitis
- Chronic progression — Intraocular lymphoma
- HIV-positive — see figure 7

FIGURE 5: Chorioretinitis

2.4 White-dot syndromes (Figure 6)

All diseases which go hand-in-hand with whitish-yellow, punctate fundus changes are grouped under the 'white-dot syndrome'.

The presence of vasculitis signals the possible presence of birdshot retinopathy. The case history is helpful only in sympathetic ophthalmia. Exudative detachment is typical of the Vogt-Koyanagi-Harada syndrome (as well as pars planitis without white spots). All these diseases can develop unilaterally or bilaterally, but the changes remain unilateral in diffuse unilateral subacute neuroretinitis. Even though the cellular infiltration of the anterior chamber or the vitreous depends on the status of inflammation, there is no anterior chamber or vitreous inflammation in the histoplasmosis syndrome or acute retinal pigment epitheliitis. It is noteworthy that some of the syndromes occur with predilection in young women.

- Vasculitis — Birdshot retinopathy
- Trauma/History of surgery — Sympathetic ophthalmia
- Exudative detachment — Vogt-Koyanagi-Harada syndrome
- Unilateral — DUSN
- No AC or vitreous inflammation
  - Histoplasmosis
  - Acute retinal pigment epitheliitis
- AC and vitreous inflammation
  - Multifocal chorioretinitis with panuveitis
  - Uveitis with subretinal fibrosis
  - APMPPE
  - Birdshot retinopathy
  - Sympathetic ophthalmia
  - Vogt-Koyanagi-Harada syndrome
- Vitreous inflammation alone
  - Multiple evanescent white dot syndrome
  - Multifocal choroiditis with panuveitis
  - Uveitis with subretinal fibrosis
  - Birdshot retinopathy
  - Serpiginous chorioretinitis
  - Diffuse unilateral subacute neuroretinitis
  - Sympathetic ophthalmia
- Predominantly younger women
  - Uveitis with subretinal fibrosis
  - Multiple evanescent white dot syndrome
  - Multifocal choroiditis with panuveitis

FIGURE 6: White-dot syndromes

2.5 Retinitis (Figure 7)

Under certain conditions, a connection can be drawn between the basic disease and the pathogenesis of retinitis. Clinical signals can be of help in AIDS-related retinitis.

Especially in the case of elderly patients and those with slow progression, one must always think of an intraocular lymphoma.

- Prior VZV infections — VZV
- Malignancies, immunosuppressive therapy — HSV, VZV
- Status post-transplantation — CMV (HSV, VZV)
- Intraocular lymphoma
- Trypanosomiasis
- In childhood
  - HSV
  - Subacute sclerosing panencephalitis

HIV+

- Encephalitis
  - Toxoplasmosis, cryptococcosis
  - Histoplasmosis
- Dermatosis — Lues
- Choroiditis
  - Pneumocystis carinii
  - Histoplasmosis
- Endophthalmitis
  - Bacillus cereus, Candida, other fungal infections
  - Staphylococcus epidermidis
- Acute progression — HSV, VZV, lues, toxoplasmosis
- Chronic progression — CMV
- Unilateral — Toxoplasmosis, lues, intraocular lymphoma
- Bilateral — CMV, HSV, VZV, toxoplasmosis, intraocular lymphoma
- Hemorrhages
  - Frequent — CMV
  - Occasional — HSV, VZV
  - Rare — Toxoplasmosis, lues, candida

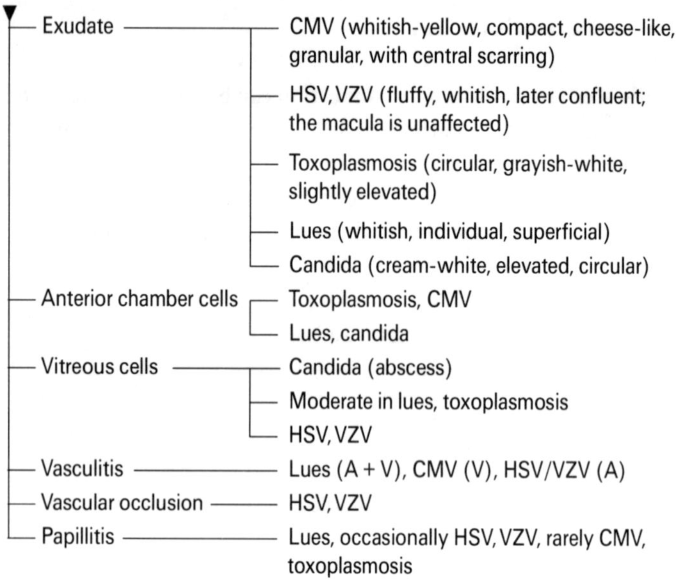

FIGURE 7: Retinitis and AIDS-related retinitis (A: arteries; V: veins)

2.6 **Vasculitis** (Figure 8)

Vasculitis is best differentiated by focussing the search on chorioretinitis or retinitis. Only in scattered cases is vascular occlusion present. In some cases, the disease leads in the long run to a tendency toward arterial or venous involvement.

- Chorioretinitis
  - White dots
    - Birdshot retinopathy
    - MEWD syndrome
    - Sarcoidosis
    - Serpiginous chorioiditis
    - VKH syndrome
    - Sympathetic ophthalmia
  - Behçet's disease
- Retinitis
  - Arteries
    - HSV, VZV
    - Toxoplasmosis
  - Veins
    - CMV, Lues, Behcet's disease
- Occlusion
  - SLE
  - Anti-phospholipid syndrome
  - Behçet's disease
  - Polyarteritis nodosa
  - Bacterial endophthalmitis
  - Rift valley fever
  - Rocky Mountain spotted fever
  - Eales' disease
- Arteries
  - Lues
  - Dermatomyositis
  - SLE
  - Polychondritis
  - Giardiasis
- Veins
  - Sarcoidosis
  - Multiple sclerosis
  - HLA-A 29+ — Birdshot retinopathy
  - Tuberculosis
  - Intermediate uveitis
  - APMPPE
- Arteries and veins
  - All diseases listed under 'arteries'
  - Kawasaki's disease
  - Thromboangiitis obliterans
  - Churg-Strauss syndrome
  - Whipple's disease

FIGURE 8: Vasculitis

2.7 Uveitis and arthritis (Figure 9)

The precise localization of arthritis can on occasion lead to a diagnosis; often, however, the presence of arthritis is only a sign of a systemic disease which underlies the uveitis and must be evaluated together with the overall clinical picture.

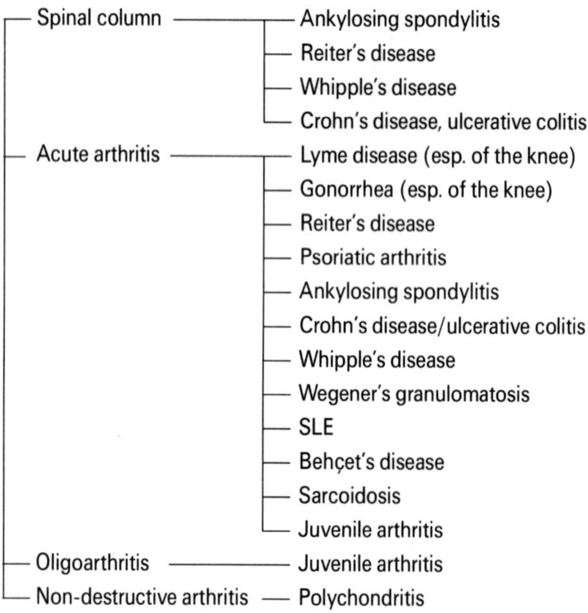

FIGURE 9: Uveitis and arthritis

2.8 Uveitis and lung involvement (Figure 10)

In addition to sarcoidosis and tuberculosis, the combination of lung disease and uveitis suggests other rare diseases.

- Sarcoidosis
- Tuberculosis
- Wegener's granulomatosis
- Allergic granulomatosis
- Coccidioidomycosis
- Kawasaki's disease
- Metastases
- Echinococcosis
- Dermatomyositis

FIGURE 10: Uveitis with lung involvement

2.9 Uveitis and skin diseases (Figure 11)

Nearly all clinical pictures which end in uveitis can be accompanied by skin changes. These may be specific (as in lues) or nonspecific (as in erythema nodosum or vitiligo). The presence of manifestations affecting other organs can lead to a very precise diagnosis here.

- Erythema nodosum
  - Behçet's disease
  - Sarcoidosis
  - SLE
  - Crohn's disease/Ulcerative colitis
  - Coccidioidomycosis
  - Leprosy
- Arthritis
  - SLE
  - Behçet's disease
  - Gonorrhea
  - Sarcoidosis
  - Psoriasis
  - Wegener's granulomatosis
  - Reiter's disease

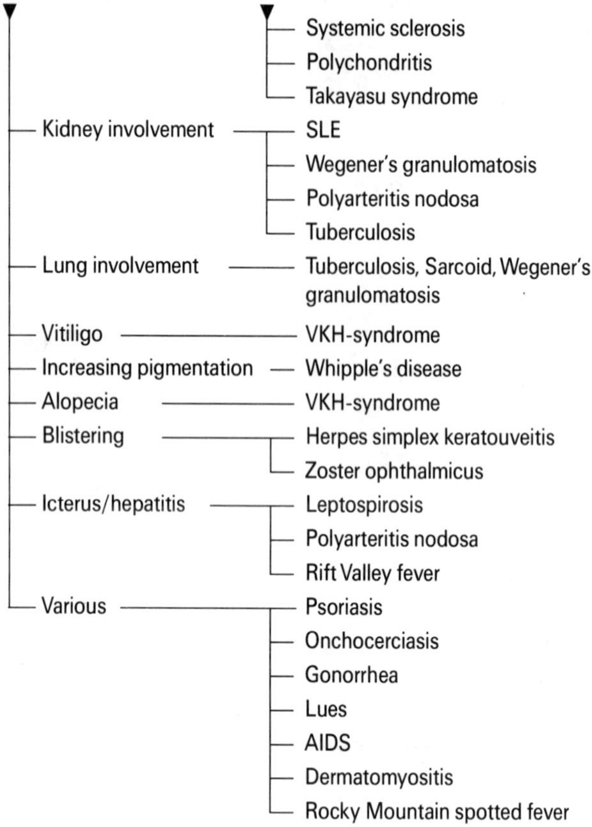

FIGURE 11: Uveitis and skin disease

2.10 Uveitis and CNS involvement (Figure 12)

CNS involvement in uveitis is often non-specific. Whereas some symptoms make their appearance in a prodromal stage (e.g. in APMPPE), permanent changes can substantiate the tentative diagnosis (e.g. in Behçet's disease, VKH syndrome).

- Meningoencephalitis/meningitis
  - Leptospirosis
  - Brucellosis
  - Congenital toxoplasmosis
  - Cryptococcosis
  - VKH syndrome
  - Behçet's disease
  - HSV
  - Lyme disease
  - Whipple's disease
  - Rift Valley fever
- Paralyses
  - Multiple sclerosis
  - SLE
  - Leprosy
  - Wegener's granulomatosis
  - Lues
  - Polyarteritis nodosa
  - Systemic sclerosis
  - Sarcoidosis
  - Churg-Strauss syndrome
  - Trypanosomiasis (sleeping sickness)
  - APMPPE
  - Sympathetic ophthalmia
  - Intraocular lymphoma
  - Subacute sclerosing panencephalitis
  - Toxoplasmosis
  - AIDS
  - VZV
  - Cysticercosis
  - Echinococcosis
  - Mucocutaneous lymph node syndrome

FIGURE 12: Uveitis with CNS involvement

2.11 Uveitis and kidney involvement (Figure 13)

In addition to various other infectious diseases, vasculitis is particularly liable to cause kidney involvement (glomerulonephritis). The combination of interstitial nephritis and anterior uveitis is characteristic for the TINU syndrome.

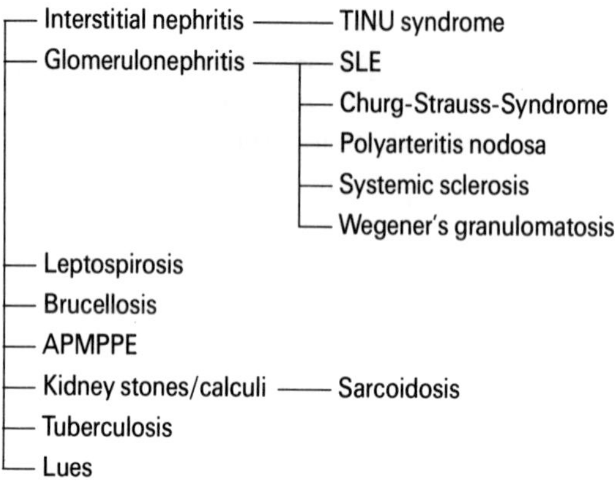

FIGURE 13: Uveitis with kidney involvement

2.12 Uveitis and involvement of the gastrointestinal tract (Figure 14)

Apart from exotic clinical pictures which can be differentiated by the clinical history, any involvement of the gastrointestinal tract should direct attention to Crohn's disease, ulcerative colitis, Whipple's disease, and polyarteritis nodosa.

- Behçet's disease
- Crohn's disease / ulcerative colitis
- Reiter's disease
- Whipple's disease
- Sarcoidosis
- Polyarteritis nodosa
- Amoebiasis
- Giardiasis
- Mucocutaneous lymph node syndrome

FIGURE 14: Uveitis with involvement of the gastrointestinal tract

- Anterior uveitis
  - Uveitis in juvenile arthritis (2 - 10)*
  - Tuberculosis
  - Sarcoidosis
  - Lyme disease
- Intermediate uveitis
  - Sarcoidosis
  - Tuberculosis
  - Mucocutaneous lymph node syndrome
  - Lyme disease
- Chorioretinitis
  - Toxoplasmosis
  - Toxocara (0 - 10)
  - Tuberculosis
  - Rubella (0 - 2)
  - Lues (0 - 2)
  - Leukemia (2 - 10)
  - Histoplasmosis (10 - 20)
  - APMPPE (10 - 20)
  - Behçet's disease
- Retinitis
  - HSV (0 - 2)
  - Subacute sclerosing panencephalitis (2 - 10)
  - CMV, HIV-retinopathy

FIGURE 15: Uveitis/retinitis in childhood

* The numbers in parentheses indicate the predominant age of manifestation.

2.13 **Uveitis in childhood** (Figure 15)

The differential diagnosis of uveitis in children is more clearly defined. Precise localization together with the possible presence of other symptoms will normally lead to correct diagnosis.

2.14 **Postoperative uveitis** (Figure 16)

Postoperative uveitis or endophthalmitis may be rooted in exogenous bacterial infection (particularly after cataract surgery) or damage to the lens (lens-induced uveitis) or in sympathetic ophthalmia (e.g. after vitrectomy).

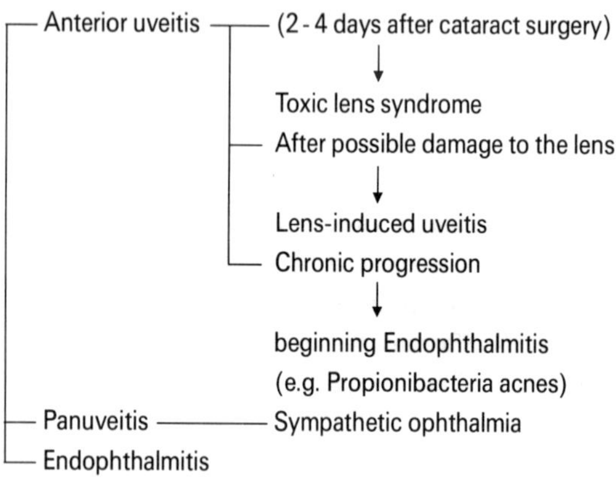

FIGURE 16: Postoperative uveitis

3. Special clinical entities

The classification of the following special clinical pictures is based initially on the localization of inflammation (anterior uveitis, posterior uveitis with the White-dot syndromes, retinitis). Retinitis, classified according to the pathogenic microorganisms, is discussed only briefly here, since it usually behaves differently from uveitis caused by the same pathogen. Where individual pathogens are also capable of triggering other forms of uveitis (e.g. herpes simplex virus), reference is made to retinitis.

This is followed by a classification according to the viral, parasitic and bacterial pathogens which lead to different forms of uveitis. Thereafter, those systemic disorders are listed which usually cause vasculitis but often other forms of retinopathy as well. Finally, postoperative uveitis and the so-called 'Masquerade' syndromes, are described.

All these clinical pictures are presented according to a uniform sequence of topics: a brief presentation of etiologic, histologic, immunopathologic, epidemiologic and other generalized information is followed by a description of systemic changes. Knowledge of not only these symptoms but also their consequences is of great importance for the ophthalmologist, since it assists him in his differential diagnosis.

This is followed by a description of the ocular changes. Here too, the whole array of diseases discussed in the literature is covered, since an overview of ophthalmologic findings can help in precisely allocating the clinical picture; however, only those changes which accompany uveitis are discussed in greater detail.

The most important tools for describing the corresponding

disorder and isolating it by differential diagnosis are given under 'Diagnosis'. Since many of the illnesses to be treated are systemic, at the beginning of this part an attempt is made to present, as far as possible, criteria for the disease which have been established to date, usually by international organizations.

The 'Remarks' occasionally made in conclusion give the author's own conclusions concerning certain controversial aspects of the disease in question.

The literature listed at the end of the discussion of a clinical picture is restricted to a few publications, preference being given to easily accessible literature.

A) Anterior uveitis

3.1 Ankylosing spondylitis (AS)

Etiology:

- Unknown
- Diverse gram-negative bacteria may act as inducers (Klebsiella pneumoniae, Shigella, Yersinia)
- Ankylosing spondylitis: HLA-B27-positive in 85-96% (vs. ca. 6% of the normal population in central Europe)
- In ankylosing spondylitis with acute anterior uveitis: ca. 95% HLA-B27-positive
- HLA-B27 appears to participate directly in the pathogenesis

General involvement:

- Arthritis of the sacroiliac joint (back pains, particularly at night; stiffness in the morning)
- Peripheral arthritis in 25% during the course of the disease
- The arthritis in HLA-B27-negative patients appears to have a milder course than in HLA-B27-positive patients
- Crohn's disease or ulcerative colitis in 10% of the patients

Ocular involvement:

- Conjunctivitis is rare
- Anterior uveitis:
  - Occasionally fibrinous or with hypopyon
  - Mostly unilateral, but can alternate
  - Mostly men are affected (80%)
  - Can be a harbinger of arthritis years ahead of time
  - Usually develops independently of arthritic activity
  - Uveitis develops in ca. 25-30% of patients with ankylosing spondylitis

Diagnosis:

- *Diagnostic criteria* (2):
  AS is confirmed if:
  - radiological confirmation of bilateral (stage 3-4) sacroiliitis is present in combination with a clinical criterion;
  - radiological confirmation of unilateral (stage 3-4) or bilateral (stage 2) sacroiliitis is present in combination with clinical criterion No. 1 or 2 and 3

  AS is possible if:
  - bilateral sacroiliitis is radiologically confirmed without clinical criteria

  Clinical criteria:
  1. Reduced mobility of the lumbar spinal column in all three degrees of free mobility
  2. History of pains in the dorsolumbar region of the spinal column
  3. Expansion of the thorax is restricted to 2.5 cm or less, measured at the level of the fourth intercostal area
- History and clinical picture
- X-ray diagnosis in case of pain
- Laboratory tests:
  - HLA-B27 typing
  - Rheumatoid factor negative
  - ANA negative

Remarks:

Uveitis displays the same characteristics in ankylosing spondylitis as in HLA-B27-positive patients without systemic disease.

Literature:

1. *Beckingsdale AB, Davies J, Gibson JL:* Acute anterior uveitis, ankylosing spondylitis, back pain and HLA-B27. Brit J Ophthalmol 68: 741-745, 1984
2. *Bennet PH, Burch TA:* New York symposium on population studies in the rheumatic diseases. New diagnostic criteria. Bull Rheum Dis 17: 453, 1967
3. *Linssen A, Rothava A, Valkenburg HA, et al.:* The lifetime cumulative incidence of acute anterior uveitis in a normal population and its relation to ankylosing spondylitis and histocompatibility antigen HLA-B27. Invest Ophthalmol Vis Sci 32: 2568-2578, 1991
4. *Scharf J, Scharf J, Haim T, et al.:* Clinical features of acute anterior uveitis. Am J Ophthalmol 103: 137-145, 1987

3.2 Reiter's disease

Etiology:

- Unknown
- Diverse gram-negative bacteria are suspected as inducers (e.g. Chlamydia, Yersinia, Salmonella)
- Reiter's disease: HLA-B27-positive in 50-70% (vs. ca. 6% of the normal population in central Europe)
- Men contract the disease 5 times as often as women
- HLA-B27 appears to participate directly in the pathogenesis

General involvement:

- Arthritis (94%), of the feet (79%), of the hands (71%), of the knees (68%), of the knuckles (52%), of the elbows, of the shoulders, of the hips (ca. 25%)
- Plantar fasciitis, Achilles tendinitis (ca. 35%)

- Back pain (29%)
- Sacroiliitis (19%)
- Urethritis
- Keratoderma blennorrhagica (10%), balanitis circinata (25-50%)
- Cystitis, prostatitis, epididymitis, orchitis
- Lesions of the oral mucosa, psoriasis-type rash, fingernail changes
- Diarrhea
- Cardiac involvement (10%)

Ocular involvement:
- Conjunctivitis with initial episode (in 30-60%)
- Keratitis
- Episcleritis (rare)
- Iritis, iridocyclitis (in 3-20%)
  - recurrent
  - rarely with initial episode

Diagnosis:
- *Diagnostic criteria* (3):

Infection of the gastro-intestinal or genitourinary tract with subsequent arthritis

- Clinical picture
- Laboratory tests:
  - HLA-B27 typing
  - Negative rheumatoid factor
  - Negative ANA
  - Leukocytosis
  - Elevation of serum globulins

Remarks:
Uveitis in Reiter's disease displays the same characteristics as uveitis in HLA-B27-positive patients without systemic disease.

Literature:

1. *Lee DA, Barker SM, Su WPD, et al:* The clinical diagnosis of Reiter's syndrome. Ophthalmology 93: 350–356, 1986
2. *Saari KM, Vilppula A, Lassus A, et al:* Ocular inflammation in Reiter's disease after Salmonella enteritis. Am J Ophthalmol 90: 63–68, 1980
3. *Wilkens RF, Arnett FC, Bitter T, et al:* Reiter's syndrome: evaluation of preliminary criteria for definite disease. Arthritis Rheum 24: 844–849, 1981

3.3 Psoriasis

Etiology:

- Unknown
- Associated with HLA-B27 20-30% of the time, 64% of the time in psoriasis-spondylitis

General involvement:

- Psoriasis can be very discrete (head, fingernail changes)
- Arthritis is present in ca. 5% of psoriasis patients
- Arthritis manifests itself particularly in the distal hand and ankle joints as well as the sacroiliac joint
- The treatment of psoriasis has no effect on the uveitis

Ocular involvement:

- Conjunctivitis
- Sicca-syndrome
- Cornea with marginal infiltrates
- Acute iridocyclitis:
  - Usually in psoriasis patients with arthritis
  - Usually unilateral

Diagnosis:

- History and clinical picture
- Laboratory tests: HLA-B27

Remarks:
In view of the frequency of psoriasis, a patient with psoriasis and uveitis does not automatically belong to this group.

Literature:

1. *Knox DL:* Psoriasis and intraocular inflammation. Trans Am Ophthalmol Soc 77: 210–224, 1979

3.4 Crohn's disease/ulcerative colitis

Etiology:
- Unknown
- A connection with infections (e.g. atypical Mycobacteria or Pseudomonas), nutritional habits or environmental factors is suspected
- Genetic associations (the family history is positive in 11%)
- Associations between ulcerative colitis with sacroiliitis and HLA-B27 (50–70% with sacroiliitis, 6% without it)

General involvement:
- Ulcerative colitis:
  - Diffuse ulceration of the entire colon:
    - Stomach pains, hemorrhagic diarrhea
    - Weight loss, fever
  - Complications:
    - Development of megacolon
    - Intestinal perforation
    - Development of pseudopolyps and malignant growths
  - Additional complications: hepatitis, sclerosing cholangitis, arthritis, erythema nodosum
  - 20-fold higher risk of developing ankylosing spondylitis
  - Anemia, leukocytosis, thrombocytosis, hypoproteinemia
- Crohn's disease:
  - localized granulomatous reaction (in 70%), potentially in all regions of the intestine, rarely in the stomach and esophagus as well

- Aphthous-like ulcers of the mucosa with development of fissures and fistulas
- Occasional involvement of skin, lungs, liver, kidneys and muscles

Ocular involvement:

- Cornea with marginal ulcers and infiltration
- Episcleritis, scleritis, necrotizing scleritis
- Iridocyclitis
- Vasculitis, occasionally obliterative
- Retinitis
- Panuveitis
- Orbital myositis, neuroretinitis
- Occasionally parallel intestinal and ocular inflammation
- Ocular problems in 4–10% of patients with Crohn's disease (43% when arthritis is present); only rarely with ulcerative colitis

Diagnosis:

- History and clinical picture
- X-ray
- Laboratory tests: stool, HLA-B27

Remarks:

Ocular involvement appears to signal Crohn's disease.

Literature:

1. *Duker JS, Brown GC, Brooks L:* Retinal vasculitis in Crohn's disease. Am J Ophthalmol 103: 664–668, 1987
2. *Hopkins DJ, Horan E, Burton IL, et al.:* Ocular disorders in a series of 322 patients with Crohn's disease. Br J Ophthalmol 58: 732–737, 1974
3. *Knox DL, Schachat AP, Mustonen E:* Primary, secondary and coincidental ocular complications of Crohn's disease. Ophthalmology 91: 163–173, 1984

3.5 HLA-B27-positive anterior uveitis without associated systemic diseases

Etiology:

- Unknown
- HLA-B27-positive in 43-60% (vs. ca. 6% of the normal population in central Europe)
- 2.5 times more frequent in men than in women
- The same 10-year prognosis as in HLA-B27-negative acute anterior uveitis

General involvement:

- No associated diseases (as per definition)

Ocular involvement:

- Anterior uveitis
  - The course appears to be more severe than in HLA-B27-negative patients
  - Unilateral (59%) but also alternating (38%)

Diagnosis:

- History and clinical picture for the exclusion of HLA-B27-associated diseases
- Laboratory tests: HLA-B27

Remarks:

Since patients with HLA-B27-positive anterior uveitis may later contract one of the associated diseases, regular repetition of rheumatological tests is indicated. HLA-typing, however, should only be carried out if anterior uveitis recurs frequently or severely.

Literature:

1. *Pavesio CE, Nozik RA:* Anterior and intermediate uveitis. Int Ophthalmol Clin 30: 244-251, 1990
2. *Rothova A, van Veenendaal WG, Linssen A, et al:* Clinical

features of acute anterior uveitis. Am J Ophthalmol 103: 137-145, 1987
3. *Wakefield D, Montanaro A, McCluskey P:* Acute anterior uveitis and HLA-B27. Surv Ophthalmol 36: 223-232, 1991

3.6 Anterior uveitis in juvenile arthritis

Etiology:

- Unknown, but microorganisms are suspected initiators
- Genetic component: serologically, frequent HLA-DR5

General involvement:

- Arthritis in children up to 16 years
- Oligoarthritic form:
  - Up to 4 (usually large) joints
  - Ocular involvement is typical in this form
  - Later transition to the polyarthritic form is possible
  - An early and a late form can be distinguished (the early form usually in girls; the late form mostly in boys; presently regarded as an HLA-B27-related disease)
- Polyarthritic form:
  - More than 5 large and small joints affected
  - Subfebrile temperatures, malaise
  - Involvement of the flexor tendon sheaths of the hands
  - Rarely pericarditis
  - Possible transition to the systemic form (Still's disease)
- Primary systemic form (Still's disease):
  - Intermittent high fever
  - Maculopapular exanthema
  - Lymphadenopathy, hepatosplenomegaly, pericarditis
  - Anemia, leukocytosis
  - Amyloidosis
  - Psoriasis
  - Ocular involvement rare

Ocular involvement:

- Iridocyclitis:
  - Usually bilateral
  - Chronic development of the early (2-6 years of age) oligoarthritic form
  - Acute development in the late (6-13 years of age) oligoarthritic form
  - The beginning is almost always asymptomatic (in contrast to the HLA-B27-positive form)

Diagnosis:

- History
- Clinical picture: rheumatologic consultation for classification of the clinical picture
- Laboratory tests:
  - Serologic tests for risk factors (ANA+, HLA-B27-negative, rheumatoid factor-negative)
  - ANA:
    - Positive in 50-90% in the early-onset form (HLA-B27-negative)
    - Negative in the late-onset oligoarthritic form (HLA-B27-positive).
  - Rheumatoid factor: classically negative

Remarks:

- Uveitis occasionally precedes arthritis by years (in about 10%)
- Iridocyclitis in juvenile arthritis has one of the poorest prognoses in uveitis, so that:
- the most intensive possible cooperation between ophthalmologist and pediatrician is necessary,
- ophthalmological checkups are required as follows(1):
  - every 2 months if ANA is positive
  - every 3 months if there is oligoarthritis
  - every 6 months if there is polyarticular involvement at the beginning
  - once a year if there is systemic disease at the beginning

Literature:

1. *Kanski JJ:* Screening for uveitis in juvenile chronic arthritis. Brit J Ophthalmol 73: 225-228, 1989
2. *Merriam JC, Chylack LT, Albert DM:* Early-onset pauciarticular juvenile rheumatoid arthritis. Arch Ophthalmol 101: 1085-1092, 1983
3. *Wolf MD, Lichter PR, Ragsdale CG:* Prognostic factors in the uveitis of juvenile rheumatoid arthritis. Ophthalmology 94: 1242-1248, 1987

3.7 Fuchs' heterochromic iridocyclitis

Etiology:

- Unknown
- At present, a viral origin is considered
- Scattered cases have been described subsequent to other ocular diseases (e.g. toxoplasmosis)

General involvement:

- None

Ocular involvement:

- Chronic iridocyclitis:
  - The eye tends to be white, with little pain
  - Very fine endothelial precipitates are distributed over the entire surface
  - The iris of the affected eye is discolored and indistinct
  - The affected eye is rarely more pigmented
  - There are almost never posterior synechiae
  - Subcapsular lens opacification in 85%
  - Glaucoma in 15-20% (steroid-induced?)
  - Although cataract extraction is usually uncomplicated, subsequent glaucoma can lead to major complications

Diagnosis:

- History and clinical picture

Remarks:

- In differentiating heterochromic iritis from cases of viral anterior uveitis, special attention should be given to the character of the pigment epithelium: it displays major damage after attacks of viral uveitis and may show heterochromia. The older literature should be evaluated with caution in this respect.
- A differentiation from other forms of uveitis is useful since cataract extraction in heterochromic uveitis has a particularly good prognosis, and the therapeutic plan for extraction is less demanding (cf. Volume 2).

Literature:

1. *Jones NP:* Fuchs' heterochromic uveitis: an update. Surv Ophthalmol 37: 253-272, 1993
2. *Liesegang TJ* Clinical features and prognosis in Fuchs' uveitis syndrome: Arch Ophthalmol 100: 1622-1626, 1982
3. *Saraux H, Laroch L, Le Hoang P:* Secondary Fuchs' heterochromic cyclitis: a new approach to an old disease. Ophthalmologica 190: 193-198,1985

3.8 Posner-Schlossman syndrome

Etiology:

- Unknown; a viral etiology (e.g. HSV) is thought possible

General involvement:

- None

Ocular involvement:

- Iritis or iridocyclitis, possibly also in the form of trabeculitis:
  - with secondary glaucoma and usually mild inflammation
  - usually unilateral

- with heterochromia of the iris in 15% of patients
- usually a good prognosis

Diagnosis:

- History and clinical picture
- Laboratory tests: where appropriate, analysis of anterior chamber puncture specimen for antiviral antibodies, e.g. anti-HSV (calculated with the Goldmann quotient)

Remarks:

It is likely that Posner-Schlossman's syndrome represents a heterogeneous clinical picture. No reports on histological studies of the acute phase are available.

Literature:

1. *Grehn F, Sundmacher R:* Zur Pathogenese und Therapie des Posner-Schlossman-Syndroms. In: Medikamentöse Glaukomtherapie, Krieglstein GK, Leydhecker W (Editors). JF Bergmann, Munich 1982
2. *Hollowich F:* Zur Klinik und Therapie des Posner-Schlossman-Syndroms. Klin Mbl Augenheilk 172: 736–744, 1978
3. *Posner A, Schlossman A:* Syndrome of unilateral recurrent attacks of glaucoma with cyclitic syndromes. Arch Ophthalmol 39: 517–528, 1948

3.9 Lens-induced uveitis

Etiology:

- Unknown; possibly an autoimmune disorder
- Tolerance for lens tissue is lost after trauma to the lens capsule, with consequent development of auto-antibodies and a possible granulomatous reaction with autoreactive T-cells
- Triggering factors:
  - Perforating injury
  - Retained lens material after cataract extraction

- Microtrauma of the capsule in mature cataract or after glaucoma surgery

General involvement:

- None

Ocular involvement:

- Anterior uveitis:
  - Granulomatous or non-granulomatous, probably depending on the degree of severity
  - Hypotonia of the globe is typical
  - Can reportedly develop between 24 hours and 40 years after the causative event
  - A frequent false diagnosis is sympathetic ophthalmia. However, both diseases are sometimes present in the same eye
  - Like sympathetic ophthalmia, it can lead to uveitis in both eyes. However, sympathetic ophthalmia invariably affects both eyes simultaneously, which is normally not the case in lens-induced uveitis
  - A frequent false diagnosis is postoperative endophthalmitis caused by, e.g. Propionibacterium acnes; here the demonstration of the pathogen is helpful.

Diagnosis:

- History and clinical picture
- IOP measurement
- Laboratory tests: attempted demonstration of the pathogen

Remarks:

- Postoperative lens-induced uveitis is too seldom diagnosed.
- The simultaneous presence of lens-induced uveitis and sympathetic ophthalmia indicates a similar reactive readiness of the immune system.
- Earlier, the granulomatous form was called 'Phacoanaphylaxis' and the non-granulomatous form 'phacotoxic' uveitis; how-

ever, these terms should be dropped, since they do not correspond to the pathogenetic mechanism.

Literature:

1. *Apple DJ, Mamalis N, Steinmetz RL, et al:* Phacoanaphylactic endophthalmitis associated with extracapsular cataract extraction and posterior chamber intraocular lens. Arch Ophthalmol 102: 1528–1532, 1984
2. *Easom HA, Zimmermann LE:* Sympathetic ophthalmia and bilateral phacoanaphylaxis. Arch Ophthalmol 72: 9–15, 1964
3. *v. Domarus D, Hinzpeter EN, Naumann G:* Klinik der 'Endophthalmitis phacoanaphylactica'. Klin Mbl Augenheilk 166: 637–644, 1975

3.10 Leptospirosis

Etiology:

- Direct action of leptospires is likely
- Infection through contact with contaminated water (e.g. urine of infected animals), soil, vegetation, or infected animals
- Typically endemic

General involvement:

- Incubation period: 1–2 weeks
- Leptospires are found in blood and CSF
- Acute onset like that of influenzal infection
- Occasional icterus, meningitis, kidney involvement

Ocular involvement:

- Anterior uveitis, often bilateral
- Rarely choroiditis
- Uveitis appears several days, even up to a year after an influenza-like prodromal stage
- Rarely involvement of the optic nerve

Diagnosis:

- History (travel, profession)
- Clinical picture
- Laboratory tests:
  - Direct demonstration of the pathogen:
    - Only in the first days of the disease
    - In blood, CSF, thereafter in urine
  - Demonstration of antibodies:
    - Especially successful if the serotypes present in the endemic area (approx. 150 are known) have already been identified (agglutination test)
    - Screening test: complement fixation reaction; however, this is negative after 3-5 months

Remarks:

The possibility of leptospirosis should be considered in high-risk patients even when there are no typical systemic symptoms. Bilateral development is particularly conspicuous; it is otherwise not common in anterior uveitis.

Literature:

1. *Barkay S, Garzozi H:* Leptospirosis and uveitis. Ann Ophthalmol 16: 164-168, 1984
2. *Gutman I, Walsh JB, Knapp AB:* Cotton-wool spots as a sign in leptospirosis. Ophthalmologica 187: 133-136, 1983
3. *Weder W:* Beobachtungen bei Leptospirosenuveitis. Klin Mbl Augenheilk 158: 330-338, 1971

3.11 Brucellosis

Etiology:

- Either direct action of Brucellae or an immunologic reaction induced by Brucellae
- Infection through contact with affected animals. High-risk groups: farmers, butchers

General involvement:

- Incubation period: 10–21 days
- Influenza-like prodromal stage
- Lymphadenopathy, splenomegaly, hepatomegaly
- Occasionally high fever, arthritis, bacterial endocarditis, orchitis, meningoencephalitis, and kidney involvement

Ocular involvement:

- Anterior uveitis
- Disseminated chorioretinitis
- Probably rarely a cause of uveitis

Diagnosis:

- History (profession, travel)
- Clinical picture
- Laboratory tests:
  - Direct demonstration: via blood cultures
  - Demonstration of antibodies
    - In the agglutination test, a fourfold rise of the titer of IgM within 1-4 weeks indicates a fresh infection
    - The test may yield negative results

Remarks:

Since brucellosis is very unusual, ocular involvement will rarely be suspected. When brucellosis is present, however, the case history and systemic manifestations should indicate it clearly. Brucellosis seems to be almost eradicated thanks to strict food-preparation and meat-handling procedures.

Literature:

1. *Poletti J, Poletti A, Larmande A:* Diagnostic and therapeutic problems in brucellosis uveitis. Med Trop 41: 523–525, 1991
2. *Rolando I, Carbone A, Haro D, Gotuzzo E, Carillo C:* Retinal detachment in chronic brucellosis. Am J Ophthalmol 99: 733–734, 1985

3. *Tabbarra KF, Al Kassimi H:* Ocular brucellosis. Br J Ophthalmol 74: 249-250, 1990

3.12 Gonorrhea

Etiology:

- Direct action of gonococci or immune mechanisms triggered by them

General involvement:

- Urethritis (25%)
- Following hematogenous spread (1-3%)
- Gonococcal arthritis-dermatitis syndrome:
  - febrile arthritis (knee)
  - papular, petechial, hemorrhagic or necrotic skin changes (65%)

Ocular involvement:

- Purulent conjunctivitis with keratitis
- Anterior uveitis (probably rare)
- Metatastic endophthalmitis (very rare)

Diagnosis:

- History
- Clinical picture
- Laboratory tests: direct demonstration of the pathogen

Remarks:

It is likely that Reiter's disease is at the root of most cases of GU-tract-associated anterior uveitis, even when gonococcal infection can be demonstrated.

Literature:

1. *Ullman S, Roussel RJ, Forster RK:* Gonococcal keratoconjunctivitis. Surv Ophthalmol 32: 199-208, 1987

3.13 Anterior uveitis in tubulo-interstitial nephritis (TINU syndrome)

Etiology:

- Unknown
- Possibly triggered by drugs (e.g. non-steroidal anti-inflammatory agents)
- Mostly in women
- No apparent age preference (contrary to earlier opinions)

General involvement:

- Symptoms of acute interstitial nephritis:
  - Febrile infection, nausea, tiredness
  - Side pains, stomach pains
  - Pyuria, elevated creatinine, often massive ESR elevation
- Acute renal failure is possible
- Histology: granulomatous or non-granulomatous infiltration

Ocular involvement:

- Conjunctivitis
- Anterior uveitis (often bilateral)
- Intraretinal bleeding
- Uveitis develops prior to or several months after the onset of the interstitial nephritis

Diagnosis:

- History (drugs, previous kidney disease)
- Clinical picture
- Laboratory tests:
  - Renal function (creatinine, creatinine clearance if there is suspicion of malfunction, urea, urinalysis)
  - Blood count (ESR)
- Precise differential diagnosis in relation to other diseases associated with kidney involvement

Remarks:

- The syndrome is more frequent than currently reported
- It is possible that the etiology is not uniform
- Careful examination of the prior drug history appears appropriate

Literature:

1. *Burnier M, Jaeger P, Campiche M, Wauters JP:* Idiopathic acute interstitial nephritis and uveitis in the adult. Am J Nephrol 6: 312–315, 1986
2. *Rosenbaum JT:* Bilateral anterior uveitis and interstitial nephritis. Am J Ophthalmol 105: 534–537, 1988
3. *Vanhaesebrouck P, Carton D, DeBel C, et al.:* Acute tubulo-interstitial nephritis and uveitis syndrome (TINU syndrome). Nephron 40: 418–422, 1985

B) Posterior uveitis

3.14 Toxoplasmosis

Etiology:

- Human infection through the uptake of oocysts (in feces) or of Toxoplasma cysts (in meat)
- Trophozoites multiply and infect healthy cells after cell rupture
- Ocular changes probably result for the most part from the secondarily initiated immune mechanisms, possibly also from auto-immune mechanisms, particularly when toxoplasma cysts rupture
- Live Toxoplasma pathogens are apparently capable of misleading the defenses of the immune system
- Contamination is especially common in warm climates (about 70% in Germany)
- Ocular involvement in combination with acquired toxoplasmosis is probably very rare; ocular involvement appears to have a frequency of about 50–70% in congenital infection

General involvement:

- Congenital form (affinity for CNS):
  - Severe clinical picture with high mortality
  - Meningoencephalitis, cramps, intracerebral calcification, hydrocephalus, vomiting, fever
  - Splenomegaly, hepatitis, hepatomegaly, lymphadenopathy, anemia
  - Diarrhea, pneumonia
- Acquired form (affinity for the lymphatic system):
  - Lymphadenopathy, hepatosplenomegaly, lymphocytosis
  - Encephalitis, personality changes
  - Pneumonia, polymyositis, maculopapular exanthema
  - Cardiac and renal involvement is also possible
  - Can end fatally in immunocompromised patients due to CNS involvement

Ocular involvement:

- Recurrent focal retinochoroiditis, retinitis, panuveitis
- Congenital toxoplamosis:
  - Fluffy, light-colored satellite spots with adjacent scar (localized recurrence)
  - Usually near the posterior pole (macula)
  - Rarely with intraretinal bleeding
  - Massive vitreous and anterior chamber reactions are typical
  - Vasculitis in the vicinity of the spot
  - Subretinal neovascularization
  - Unilaterally active, but often with bilateral scars
  - Microphthalmia, cataract, and optic nerve atrophy have also been described
  - Juxtapapillary involvement, sometimes isolated (in most instances probably the syndrome designated as 'Jensen's disease')
  - Small white spots in the inner retinal layers are also possible; these are part of the 'White-dot syndrome' and are primarily associated with only mild vitreous irritation or none at all (2)

- Acquired toxoplasmosis:
  - The rate of incidence is still very much a matter of controversy, but it appears to develop in combination with toxoplasmosis-encephalitis
  - Has been reported after blood transfusions
  - Satellite spots as in congenital toxoplasmosis
- Retinitis under immune suppression:
  - During immunosuppressive therapy, AIDS (cf. Chap. 3.26)
  - Can develop as the first manifestation of an AIDS infection
  - Usually more pronounced vitreous flare than in CMV, HSV or VZV-retinitis
  - Often more than one active spot is visible
  - Can be active in both eyes

Diagnosis:

- Clinical picture: may be very typical
- Fluorescein angiography:
  - Early phase: blockade of the fluorescein
  - Late phase: leakage from the active spot
- Laboratory tests:
  - Determination of specific antibodies
    - Immunofluorescence test
    - ELISA: Determination of IgM indicates that infection has subsided only a short time ago
    - Negative test results are an unequivocal indication that no toxoplasmosis is present; positive test results are inconclusive because of the prevalence of contamination

Remarks:

- Tests for antibodies against toxoplasmosis are meaningful only in retinochoroiditis. However, antibodies are then nearly always found.
- Because of the prevalence of exposure in the general population, demonstration of anti-toxoplasmosis antibodies is not proof of toxoplasmosis; their absence, on the other hand,

nearly always eliminates the possibility of toxoplasmosis. An exception to this is found in immunosuppressed patients, since they may be no longer capable of adequately developing antibodies.

- Many important questions about the prevalence of toxoplasmosis remain unsolved, such as the significance of acquired toxoplasmosis and the question whether siblings born after a toxoplasmosis-infected baby are still protected. Family studies in Brazil cast doubt on this hypothesis and indicate acquired toxoplasmosis as an important cause of ocular disease.

Literature:

1. *Akstein RB, Wilson LA, Teutsch SM:* Acquired toxoplasmosis. Ophthalmology 89: 1299-1301, 1982
2. *Deft BH, Gass JD:* Outer retinal layer toxoplasmosis. Graefes Arch Clin Exp Ophthalmol 224: 78-82, 1986
3. *Jabs DA:* Ocular toxoplasmosis. Int Ophthalmol Clin 30: 264-270, 1990
4. *Rothova A, van Knapen F, Baarsma GS, et al.:* Serology in ocular toxoplasmosis. Br J Ophthalmol 70: 615-622, 1986
5. *Yeo JH, Jakobiec FA, Iwamoto T, et al.:* Opportunistic toxoplasmic retinochoroiditis following chemotherapy for systemic lymphoma. A light and electron microscopic study. Ophthalmology 90: 885-898, 1983

3.15 Toxocara

Etiology:

- The eggs of Toxocara canis are eliminated by dogs and transferred to humans (food, children's sandboxes)
- The larvae thereafter mature in the intestinal tract and induce organ manifestations from there
- Development of granuloma in the eye indicates a T-cell-mediated immune reaction against larvae localized in the choroid; this can also lead to necrosis

General involvement:

- Visceral larva migrans (VLM) disease:
  - Contracted in the 1st to 4th year of life
  - Fever, coughing, nausea, abdominal pains with diarrhea
  - Hepatosplenomegaly, involvement of the liver, lungs, and CNS
  - Eosinophilia, leukocytosis, and hypergammaglobulinemia
  - No ocular involvement at this stage

Ocular involvement:

- Retinochoroidal granuloma, endophthalmitis
- Only in conjunction with ocular toxocariasis, which can appear without or years after systemic disease
- Macular form:
  - Whitish, round granuloma
  - Subretinal bleeding, waxy exudate or even exudative detachment are possible
  - Vitreous reaction is usually mild
  - Usually in children
- Peripheral form:
  - Peripheral granuloma, usually located inferiorly
  - Moderate to massive vitreous reaction
  - Vitreous traction, possibly traction with retinal detachment
- Endophthalmitis:
  - Densified vitreous
  - Granuloma is found sonographically
  - Pronounced anterior chamber flare
  - Possible development of a retrolental membrane
  - Possible calcification as in retinoblastoma
- Rarely optic nerve neuritis

Diagnosis:

- The history is occasionally helpful (contact with dogs)
- Clinical picture: development of granulomas

Laboratory tests:

- Eosinophilia: is almost always confined to the aqueous or vitreous puncture specimens
- Demonstration of antibodies (ELISA):
  - Sensitivity 95%, specificity 72% with a titer of 1:2
  - Sensitivity 85%, specificity 94% with a titer of 1:16
  - In the anterior chamber or vitreous puncture specimen, the antibody titer is higher than in the serum

Remarks:

In the presence of leukokoria, retinoblastoma must be considered.

Literature:

1. *Maguire AM, Green WR, Michels RG, Erozan YS:* Recovery of intraocular Toxocara canis by pars plana vitrectomy. Ophthalmology 97: 675–680, 1990
2. *Shields JA:* Ocular toxocariasis. A review. Surv Ophthalmol 28: 361–381, 1984

3.16 Histoplasmosis

Etiology:

- Evoked by inhalation of spores of the fungus Histoplasma capsulatum
- Endemic ocular symptoms are practically confined to the Ohio-Mississippi area
- Histopathology: granulomatous and non-granulomatous changes with central necrosis
- It is not known how Histoplasma capsulatum leads to choroiditis; up to the present, demonstration with tissue biopsies has succeeded only in the case of immunosuppressed patients, explaining the continued use of the term 'Presumed Ocular-Histoplasmosis-Syndrome'

General involvement:

- After inhalation of the fungus spores

- Fungemia
- Mediastinitis, lymphadenopathy
- Pericarditis, pneumonia, meningitis
- The course of infection is asymptomatic in 99%

Ocular involvement:

- Multifocal choroiditis:
  - Usually peripheral, therefore asymptomatic
  - Leaves behind 'histospots', i.e. depigmented, atrophic scars 0.2–0.7 optic disc diameter in size, with an occasional central pigment spot
  - Later the spots are usually peripapillary as well
  - Exudative hemorrhagic maculopathy (63%); this can ensue years later
  - Subretinal neovascularization membrane
  - Occasional vitreous hemorrhage
  - Ultimately: disciform macular atrophy
  - Continued development of 'histospots'
  - The vitreous is invariably free of cells
- Choroiditis in immunosuppressed patients (cf. Chap 3.26)

Diagnosis:

- Clinical picture: typical
- Laboratory tests:
  - Antibody demonstration (complement fixation reaction)
    - Antibodies are present in cases of primary infection, but only in 30% of patients with maculopathy
  - HLA-B27 appears to be more frequent in patients with macular involvement
- Histoplasmin skin test:
  - Too many false-negative results
  - Can lead to activation of dormant or not yet visible spots

Remarks:

Except in endemic areas of the USA, the diagnosis 'Histoplasmosis syndrome' should be given only with great caution.

A clinical picture described outside the USA is always characterized by a negative skin test. Its etiology is unknown, and there is no connection with endemic histoplasmosis areas (1).

Literature:

1. *Saraux H, Pelosse B, Guigui A:* Choroitide multifocale interne pseudohistoplasmose. Forme européenne de l'histoplasmose présumée américaine. J Fr Ophtalmol 9: 645–651, 1986
2. *Schlaegel TF, Weber JC, Hebbeston E:* Presumed ocular histoplasmosis. Am J Ophthalmol 63: 919–925, 1960
3. *Watzke RC, Claussen RW:* The long term course of multifocal choroiditis (presumed ocular histoplasmosis). Am J Ophthalmol 91: 750–760, 1981

C) White-dot syndromes

Numerous inflammatory changes of the retina and the choroid occur in conjunction with whitish, round changes, at least for a certain period of time; in addition to the inflammatory changes already described at length (histoplasmosis, sarcoidosis), these changes can be grouped together under the term 'White-dot syndrome'.

3.17 Birdshot retinochoroidopathy

Etiology:

- Unknown
- Possibly the human equivalent of experimentally induced auto-immune uveitis, in which the retinal S-molecule represents the autoantigen
- HLA-A29 is positive in 80–96% of patients
- Primary inflammation of the choroidal vessels is possible

General involvement:

- None

Ocular involvement:

- White to cream-colored circular lesions, concentrated at the posterior pole
- Vitreous cells; the anterior chamber is usually free of irritation
- There is almost always concomitant vasculitis
- Rarely, subretinal neovascularization at the posterior pole
- Optic nerve atrophy
- Typically bilateral

Diagnosis:

- Laboratory tests: HLA-A29
- Fluorescein angiography:
  - Early phase: Only moderate staining of the white spots.
  - Late phase: Possible mild hyperfluorescence in the area of the spots

Remarks:

In contrast to some other diseases of the fundus which belong to the White-dot syndrome, the prognosis in birdshot retinopathy is unfavorable. If there is chorioretinitis with round spots together with positive HLA-A29, birdshot retinopathy should be assumed, at least as a working diagnosis. HLA-A29 is also found with markedly greater frequency in vasculitis of unknown origin than in the healthy population (1).

Literature:

1. *Bloch-Michel E, Frau E:* Birdshot retinochoroidopathy and HLA-A29+ and HLA-A29- idiopathic retinal vasculitis: comparative study of 56 cases. Can J Ophthalmol 26: 361-366, 1991
2. *Gass JDM:* Vitiliginous chorioretinitis. Arch Ophthalmol 99: 1778-1787, 1981
3. *Nussenblatt RB, Mittal KK, Ryan SJ, et al.:* Birdshot retinochoroidopathy associated with HLA-A29 antigen and immune responsiveness to retinal S-antigen. Am J Ophthalmol 94: 147-158, 1982

4. *Priem H, Oosterhuis JA:* Birdshot chorioretinopathy: clinical characteristics and evolution. Br J Ophthalmol 72: 646–659, 1988
5. *Ryan SJ, Maumenee AE:* Birdshot retinochoroidopathy. Am J Ophthalmol 89: 31–45, 1980

3.18 Acute posterior multifocal placoid pigment epitheliopathy (APMPPE)

Etiology:

- Unknown; viral?
- Adenovirus type 5 was isolated in a throat smear from a patient with a head cold
- With regard to the pathogenesis, it is generally assumed that APMPPE most likely occurs in the context of choroidal vasculitis and secondary damage to the retinal pigment epithelium
- The patients are mostly young (20–30 years of age)

General involvement:

- Often in combination with mild viral infections
- Scattered reports exist of nephritis, erythema nodosum and cerebral vasculitis

Ocular involvement:

- Usually bilateral, multifocal, yellowish, round, plaque-like changes
- Begins at the posterior pole, does not go beyond the equator
- Runs its course at the level of the pigment layer
- Mild vitreous reaction, no anterior chamber reaction
- Occasional papillitis; rarely, cystoid macular edema
- Very rarely a subretinal neovascularization membrane
- Probably self-limiting; vision improves within a few weeks
- The scars are soft and not clearly circumscribed
- Recurrences are possible
- The prognosis is very good

Diagnosis:

- Fluorescein angiography:
  - For differentiation from other white-dot syndromes
  - For follow-ups
  - Early phase: Hypofluorescence is typical (filling defects of the choriocapillaris or blockade due to the RPE)
  - Late phase: Hyperfluorescence and leakage (diagnostic differentiation from 'Multiple evanescent white-dot syndrome')
- Electrophysiology: the EOG shows clear changes in the acute phase

Remarks:

In view of the good prognosis, problems arise only very rarely in APMPPE.

Literature:

1. *Deutman AF, Lion F:* Choriocapillaris nonperfusion in acute multifocal placoid pigment epitheliopathy. Am J Ophthalmol 84: 652-657, 1977
2. *Gass JDM:* Acute posterior multifocal placoid pigment epitheliopathy. Arch Ophthalmol 80: 177-185, 1968
3. *Kottow A:* Akute Pigmentepitheliopathien der Netzhaut. Klin Mbl Augenheilk 176: 752-757, 1980

3.19 Acute retinal pigment epitheliitis

Etiology:

- Unknown, possibly viral
- No known sex predilection

General involvement:

- None

Ocular involvement:

- Small, dark-gray to black spots in the deep retinal layers, surrounded by a yellow ring in the acute phase
- Can develop into central serous retinopathy
- No vitreous or anterior chamber involvement
- Prognosis is good (visual improvement in 6–12 weeks)

Diagnosis:

- Fluorescein angiography:
  - Early phase: hypofluorescence with surrounding hyperfluorescence; very minor leakage
  - Late phase: hyperfluorescence, possibly signs of central serous retinopathy with marked leakage
- Electrophysiology:
  - EOG: pathologic in the acute phase
  - ERG: normal

Remarks:

It is still unclear to what extent pigment epitheliitis is a cause of central serous retinopathy. Because the prognosis is typically very good, there are no therapeutic problems.

Literature:

1. *Deutman AF:* Acute retinal pigment epitheliitis. Am J Ophthalmol 78: 571–578, 1974
2. *Friedman MW:* Bilateral recurrent acute retinal pigment epitheliitis. Am J Ophthalmol 79: 567–570, 1975
3. *Krill AE, Deutman AF:* Acute retinal pigment epitheliitis. Am J Ophthalmol 74: 193–205, 1972

3.20 Multiple evanescent white-dot syndrome (MEWDS)

Etiology:

- Unknown, possibly viral

General involvement:

- Occasionally a viral infection with mild development precedes ocular involvement

Ocular involvement:

- Multiple small (100–200 μm) white lesions in the deep retina or pigment epithelium
- White, round spots extending from the posterior pole to the middle periphery and smaller than in APMPPE
- Granular appearance of the macula is typical
- Moderate vitreous reaction without anterior chamber cells
- Occasional sheathing of retinal veins
- Occasional recurrences
- Disease of young people (average age: 28 years)
- Predominantly women (75%)
- Probably a self-limiting disease (visual recovery within 1–16 weeks)
- A connection with the syndrome of 'acute idiopathic blind spot enlargement' (AIBSE) or acute macular neuropathy (AMN) has been suggested

Diagnosis:

- Fluorescein angiography:
  - For differentiation from other white-dot syndromes
  - Early phase: hypofluorescence is typical
  - Late phase: hyperfluorescence
- Electrophysiology:
  - ERG: pathological in the acute phase
- Laboratory tests:
  - Determination of antiviral antibodies would be appropriate in case of a corresponding history. Until now, however, only elevated total IgG and IgM levels have been found in the serum; although this indicates infection, the specific antibodies have not yet been determined

Remarks:

In view of the good prognosis, there are practically no grave diagnostic problems in MEWDS. MEWDS is probably rare; however, a large number of unknown cases can be presumed because of the rapid recovery.

Literature:

1. *Aaberg TM, Campo RV, Joffe L:* Recurrences and bilaterality in the multiple evanescent white-dot syndrome. Am J Ophthalmol 100: 29–37, 1985
2. *Gass JDM, Hamed LM:* Acute macular neuroretinopathy and multiple evanescent white dot syndrome occurring in the same patient. Arch Ophthalmol 107: 189–193, 1989
3. *Jampol LM, Sieving PA, Pugh D, et al.:* Multiple evanescent white dot syndrome: I. Clinical findings. Arch Ophthalmol 102: 671–674, 1984
4. *Mamalis N, Daily MJ:* Multiple evanescent white-dot syndrome. A report of eight cases. Ophthalmology 94: 1209–1212, 1987

3.21 Serpiginous choroiditis

Etiology:

- Unknown
- The process leads to RPE atrophy and to loss of the choriocapillaris and the vascular structure of the choroid

General involvement:

- None

Ocular involvement:

- Choroiditis:
  - Gray-white, punctate spots with blurred contours, later evolving into flat, map-like edematous foci
  - Usually beginning at the posterior pole (optic disc)

- New spots begin at the margin of the old scar
- Involvement of the macula in 20%, with subretinal neovascularization membrane
- Occasionally vitreous and possible anterior chamber reaction
- Occasionally vasculitis with bleeding
- Usually bilateral, but years may pass before it appears in the second eye
- Poor prognosis if the macula is involved

Diagnosis:

- Clinical picture
- Electrophysiology:
  - Lowered EOG in the affected and non-affected eye
- Fluorescein angiography:
  - Early phase: hypofluorescence at the active margins
  - Late phase: hyperfluorescence at the active margins

Remarks:

Since histologic and immunohistopathologic studies of the acute stage of this disease are still unavailable, it remains unclear whether this may be a degenerative rather than an inflammatory process; this would at least explain why the disease appears to follow its own laws in the face of therapy.

Literature:

1. *Chisholm RR, Gass JDM, Hutton WL:* The late stage of serpiginous (geographic) choroiditis. Am J Ophthalmol 82: 343-357, 1976
2. *Mansour AM, Jampol LM, Packo KH, Hrisomalos NF:* Macular serpiginous choroiditis. Retina 8: 125-131, 1988
3. *Schatz H, Maumenee AE, Patz A:* Geographic helicoid peripapillary choroidopathy: clinical presentation and fluorescein angiographic findings. Trans Am Acad Ophthalmol Otolaryngol 78: 747-761, 1974

3.22 Sympathetic ophthalmia

Etiology:

- Unknown
- A possible autoimmune reaction against a retinal antigen is often discussed
- Mediated by T-cells
- Histopathology: granulomatous, but occasionally also non-granulomatous reaction of the uvea, with peripheral location as Dalen-Fuchs' nodules between the pigment epithelium and Bruch's membrane; on rare occasions the choriocapillaris is involved
- Induced by:
  - 0.2-0.5% of penetrating injuries
  - 0.01-0.06% of vitrectomies
  - 0.007% of other intraocular procedures (cataract extraction, iridectomy, paracentesis, cyclodialysis, retinal detachment surgery, keratectomy)
  - YAG capsulotomy in rare cases
- Time interval: within 3 months in 70-80%, within a year after the causative event in 90%
- However: Reports exist of first appearances after 5 days and up to 66 years later

General involvement:

- The CNS is very rarely involved:
  - cells in the spinal fluid
  - impaired hearing
  - hair and skin changes
- Overlaps with Vogt-Koyanagi-Harada syndrome

Ocular involvement:

- Chronically recurring iridocyclitis (45%) with pain and photophobia
- Bilateral panuveitis (an unilateral form which has an especially mild course has been reported)

- Often granulomatous
- Gray-white, often initially peripheral choroidal spots (Dalen-Fuchs' nodules) which are round and sometimes confluent (25-45%)
- Papillitis (about 50%)
- Optic nerve atrophy (about 54%)
- Reduced ocular accommodation due to cyclitis, usually as the initial sign
- Frequently secondary glaucoma
- Retinal detachment (reported in 42% of the sympathizing eyes)
- Phacogenic uveitis (reported in 23-46%)
- There are many similarities to Vogt-Koyanagi-Harada syndrome (cf. Chap. 3.23)

Diagnosis:
- History and clinical picture
- Accommodation measurement
- Fluorescein angiography:
  - Acute stage: initial blockade due to Dalen-Fuchs' nodules, later subretinal, confluent dots with hyperfluorescence, occasionally of the retinal blood vessels as well
- In the scarring phase: window defects
- Electrophysiology:
  - Reduced amplitudes in ERG and EOG

Literature:

1. *Goto H, Rao NA:* Sympathetic ophthalmia and Vogt-Koyanagi-Harada syndrome. Int Ophthalmol Clin 30: 279-285, 1990
2. *Kraus-Mackiw E:* Prevention of sympathetic ophthalmia. State of the art 1989. Int Ophthalmol 14: 391-394, 1990
3. *Lubin JR, Albert DM, Weinstein M:* Sixty-five years of sympathetic ophthalmia. Ophthalmology 87: 109-121, 1980

3.23 Vogt-Koyanagi-Harada syndrome

Etiology:

- Unknown; a viral etiology has been suggested
- A systemic autoimmune disease is suspected which is directed against an autoantigen common to all affected organs
- The autoantigen may be a component of the melanocytes of the basement membrane
- A genetic component exists:
  Serology: HLA-DR4 in Japan in 88% of the patients (32% of controls), HLA-Dw15
- Histopathology: diffuse or localized (Dalen-Fuchs' nodules), granulomatous reaction in the uvea; can also be non-granulomatous in the chronic phase; pigment epithelial hyperplasia with clumping; infiltration of plasma cells, T-cells, later also involvement of the choriocapillaris and the retina
- The histological picture is highly reminiscent of sympathetic ophthalmia and in case of doubt hardly distinguishable
- Frequent in Japan and Brazil (8% of uveitis patients), rare in white patients
- The prognosis is variable, occasionally poor

General involvement:

- Occasionally there is a prodromal phase with headache, stiffness of the neck, pain in the orbital area, fever, encephalopathy
- In the prodromal and acute stages: contact hypersensitivity of skin and hair (72%)
- In the scarring phase: vitiligo, poliosis, e.g. of the eyebrows, eyelashes or scalp hair (63-90%), alopecia (73%)
- Inner-ear hearing impairment (75%); tinnitus, dizziness (rare)

Ocular involvement:

- Panuveitis:
  - Exudative retinal detachment or elevation with moderate, sometimes superficial RPE irregularities (hypo- or hyper-

pigmentation) or subretinal strips and lines of demarcation (Harada component)
- Multifocal choroidal spots, later confluent
- Usually massive anterior chamber reaction (56%)
- Occasional nodules in the iris stroma
- Possible subretinal and optic nerve neovascularization
- The retinal vascular system is largely unaffected
- Occasional depigmentation as a first sign, beginning in the limbus area (Sugiura's sign) 1 month after onset of the disease
- Early optic disc edema (87%) or hyperemia
- Nearly always bilateral, but not always with simultaneous onset

• Primary optic nerve neuritis

Diagnosis:

• Criteria: two symptoms should be demonstrable in each group:
  - Alopecia, poliosis, vitiligo
  - Neurologic symptoms: headache, stiff neck, encephalopathy, impaired hearing, pleocytosis in the cerebrospinal fluid
  - Uveitis: the following are typical: bilaterality, acute onset with retinal edema, fluorescein leakage at the level of the pigment epithelium, optic disc edema

• Fluorescein angiography:
  - Early phase of illness: numerous subretinal leakages
  - Later in the course: window defects, possible display of neovascularization membranes, arteriovenous anastomoses, confluent leakages

• Electrophysiologic tests:
  - ERG, EOG: a better criterion than visual acuity in some instances
  - Determination of central critical flicker frequency: differentiation between primary optic nerve involvement (frequency normally less than 20 Hz) and secondary optic nerve involvement (frequency normally above 20 Hz)

- Laboratory tests: lymphocytic pleocytosis in the cerebrospinal fluid (80%)

Literature:

1. *Beniz J, Forster DJ, Lean JS, et al.:* Variations in clinical features of the Vogt-Koyanagi-Harada Syndrome. Retina 11: 275–280, 1991
2. *Ohno S, Minakawa R, Matsuda H:* Clinical studies on Vogt-Koyanagi-Harada's disease. Jap J Ophthalmol 32: 334–343, 1988
3. *Perry HD, Font RL:* Clinical and histopathologic observations in severe Vogt-Koyanagi-Harada syndrome. Am J Ophthalmol 83: 242–254, 1977

3.24 Multifocal chorioretinitis with panuveitis

Etiology:
- Unknown
- Possibly viral (e.g. Epstein-Barr virus, cf. Chap. 3.31)
- Often similar to sarcoidosis

General involvement:
- Scattered cases of febrile illness prior to ocular involvement have been described

Ocular involvement:
- Multifocal white spots in the pigment epithelium or the choroid (as in histoplasmosis), ca. 50–200 μm in diameter, with a punched-out appearance
- The spots are partially pigmented
- Frequent peripapillary pigment changes (as in histoplasmosis)
- Mostly vitreous and anterior chamber inflammation (in contrast to histoplasmosis)
- Cystoid macular edema (14–41%)
- Rarely, subretinal neovascularization

- More women are affected than men
- Very often myopes
- Prognosis moderate to poor

Diagnosis:
- Fluorescein angiography for differential diagnosis:
  - Early hyperfluorescence of the spots (RPE defect)
  - Possible late leakage
- ERG: unremarkable or marginal

Remarks:
There is little clinical experience with this disease. It appears that the same overall picture can appear in Epstein-Barr viral infections (cf. Chap. 3.31)

Literature:

1. *Dreyer RF, Gass JDM:* Multifocal choroiditis and panuveitis: a syndrome that mimics ocular histoplasmosis. Arch Ophthalmol 102: 1776-1784, 1984
2. *Joondeph BC, Tessler HH:* Multifocal choroiditis. Int Ophthalmol Clin 30: 286-290, 1990
3. *Morgan CM, Schatz H:* Recurrent multifocal choroiditis. Ophthalmology 93: 1138-1147, 1986

3.25 Uveitis with subretinal fibrosis

Etiology:
- Unknown
- Histologically, primary damage to the choroid leads to antibody deposits above Bruch's membrane with subsequent RPE and retinal changes and fibrosis
- Described until now only in young, mostly black women

General involvement:
- None

Ocular involvement:

- Yellowish-white subretinal spots with a gliotic, fibrotic appearance
- The spots may be confluent and finally cover the entire posterior pole including the macula and the optic disc
- Massive vitreous reaction
- A mild anterior chamber reaction is possible
- Almost always bilateral

Diagnosis:

- Clinical picture:
  - Initially, typical white-dot syndrome
  - Later development of fibrosis
- Electrophysiology:
  - ERG and EOG show marked changes in the late phase
- Fluorescein angiography:
  - Early phase: choroidal blockade through fibrosis, but also hyperfluorescence
  - Late phase: window defects of the lesions

Remarks:

Little has been published on the syndrome of uveitis with subretinal fibrosis. It is quite possible that this type of uveitis represents an extreme form of uveitis which has previously been classified otherwise.

Literature:

1. *Cantrill HL, Folk JC:* Multifocal choroiditis associated with progressive subretinal fibrosis. Am J Ophthalmol 101: 170-180, 1986
2. *Kim MK, Chan CC, Belfort R, et al.:* Histopathologic and immunohistopathologic features of subretinal fibrosis and uveitis syndrome. Am J Ophthalmol 104: 15-23, 1987
3. *Palestine AG, Nussenblatt RB, Parver L, Knox D:* Progressive subretinal fibrosis and uveitis. Br J Ophthalmol 68: 667-673, 1984

D) Retinitis

3.26 Retinitis and choroiditis in AIDS

Etiology:

- Infection of CD4-positive lymphocytes (T-helper cells/inducer cells) with HIV (human immunodeficiency virus) leads, after cytolysis, to a predominance of CD8-positive T-suppressor/cytotoxic lymphocytes
- As a consequence: massive weakening of the T-cell system and, secondarily, of antibody production
- Patients at risk:
  - Homosexual and bisexual men
  - Heterosexual partners of HIV-infected persons
  - Drug addicts and prostitutes
  - Newborn children of HIV-infected mothers
  - Hemophiliacs
- Transmission: sexual contact, blood, transfusion with contaminated blood (89-100% risk of infection), via the placenta
- The type of opportunistic infection depends on the number of T-cells

General involvement:

- After infection:
  - Latency: 6 months to 12 years
  - Lymphadenopathy syndrome: painless lymph nodes which persist for 3 months and are larger than 1 cm in diameter at at least two extra-inguinal locations
  - AIDS-related complex: anorexia, weakness, fever, nocturnal sweating, diarrhea, weight loss, Kaposi's sarcoma, generalized lymphadenopathy, herpes zoster, oral candidiasis, oral leukoplakia
  - AIDS: development of opportunistic infections and neoplasms

Ocular involvement:

- Occurs in 75% of AIDS patients
- Unspecific complaints such as blurred vision, photophobia (cause usually unknown), night blindness (malabsorption of vitamin A)
- Cranial nerve paralysis, pupil malfunction, visual hallucination, motility disturbances (as possible early symptoms)
- Eyelids: molluscum contagiosum, ulcers
- Conjunctiva: microvasculopathy, subconjunctival bleeding
- Keratoconjunctivitis sicca (10–15%)
- Herpes zoster ophthalmicus as a possible first sign (cf. Chap. 3.30)
- Herpes simplex keratitis may take a more severe course, with frequent recurrences
- Bacterial and mycotic keratitis
- Neoplasms of the orbits and eyelids: Kaposi's sarcoma (in 25% of AIDS patients, with further ophthalmologic symptoms in 20%), Burkitt's lymphoma (non-Hodgkin lymphoma)
- Retinitis and choroiditis:
  - Often as a first manifestation of AIDS
  - Vitreous infiltration in retinitis as a sign of immunosuppression in HIV infection is milder than in immunocompetent patients with the same form of retinitis
  - Numerous publications have reported finding 2 or more potential retinitis pathogens in retinal biopsies of HIV-infected persons
  - Infections with the following have been described:
  - Cytomegalovirus:
    - The most frequent retinitis in AIDS (30% of AIDS patients)
    - First AIDS symptom in 2% of the patients
    - Occasionally accompanied by optic nerve neovascularization
    - Often only minimal vitreous reaction
    - Bilateral in 30%

- Most common retinitis if CD4 count is less than 60 cells/ mm^3
  - Further information: cf. Chap. 3.28
- Herpes simplex virus:
  - Occasionally preceded by HSV dermatitis
  - 30% bilateral
  - Further information: cf. Chaps. 3.27 and 3.29
- Varicella zoster virus:
  - Occasionally preceded by zoster dermatitis or zoster ophthalmicus
  - The infection is often longer and more severe than in non-HIV+ patients
  - 30% bilateral
  - Further information: cf. Chaps. 3.27 and 3.30
  - Progressive outer retinal necrosis syndrome:
    - possibly caused by VZV
    - multifocal retinal opacification
    - first seen in the outer layers
    - little inflammation
    - rapid progression, leading to total retinal necrosis
- HIV:
  - Retinitis:
    - Whether HIV itself can cause retinitis is not certain. However, HIV has been found with CMV in retinal biopsies; this is viewed at present as synergism
  - Microvasculopathy:
    - HIV can infect retinal tissue, particularly capillary, endothelial and neuroretinal tissue and thus lead to the development of cotton-wool spots; this in turn may pave the way for a CMV infection
    - Cotton-wool spots appear in 50% of AIDS patients and are usually seen along the major vessels at the posterior pole; they appear suddenly and disappear within 2 months
- Human herpes virus type 6:

  - Has been found with HIV and/or CMV in retinitis lesions
  - A possibile role in the development of retinitis is unclear
- Lues:
  - HIV-induced immunosuppression appears to increase susceptibility to new lues infections and the potential for transmission
  - Retinitis:
    - Normally in the secondary stage
    - Simultaneous neurosyphilis in 85% of patients
    - The course is more severe in AIDS, lasts longer, recurs more often, and is more difficult to treat
    - The typical primary stage of lues may fail to develop
    - The VDRL test may be negative
    - Further information: cf. Chap. 3.51
  - HIV patients should be examined for lues and lues-positive patients for HIV
- Bacillus cereus:
  - Endophthalmitis
- Staphylococcus epidermidis:
  - Endophthalmitis
- Mycobacterium avium:
  - Choroiditis
- Toxoplasma gondii:
  - Appears to be a consequence of new infection or extra-ocular dissemination
  - Associated with toxoplasmosis-encephalitis in 50%
  - Multifocal spots, unrelated to pre-existing scars
  - Occasionally found simultaneously with CMV
  - Anterior chamber involvement is usual
  - Occasionally with retinal hemorrhages or retinal detachment
  - Further information: cf. Chap. 3.14
- Pneumocystis carinii:
  - Multifocal choroidal infiltration
  - Minimal vitreous reaction

- Almost always with simultaneous pneumonia
    - Occurs under pentamidine aerosol therapy (pneumonia prophylaxis)
    - In all likelihood rare
  - Candida:
    - Retinitis is rare
    - Yellowish, mostly focal spots
    - Often surrounded by bleeding
    - Further information: cf. Chap. 3.45
  - Cryptococcus:
    - Choroiditis, less often retinitis
    - Normally combined with Cryptococcus meningitis
    - As a consequence: optic disc edema, diplopia, nystagmus, paralysis of the 6th cranial nerve, ophthalmoplegia, ptosis, optic nerve atrophy
    - Further information: cf. Chap. 3.48
  - Histoplasma capsulatum:
    - Retinitis, choroiditis, optic nerve involvement
    - Often combined with disseminated histoplasmosis
    - Further information: cf. Chap. 3.16
  - Choroiditis tuberculosa (cf. Chap. 3.49)

Diagnosis:

- History and clinical picture
- Laboratory tests:
  - HIV: Demonstration of specific antibodies:
    - ELISA: Screening; false-positive test results are possible
    - Western blot test
    - Indirect immunofluorescence
  - Retinitis:
    - CMV: Positive cultures in the vitreous puncture specimen, urine cultures
    - HSV: Sometimes positive cultures in the vitreous puncture specimen
    - VZV: Sometimes positive cultures in the vitreous puncture specimen

- Toxoplasmosis: Demonstration of serum antibodies
- Lues: Serum FTA-ABS and VDRL tests positive

Literature:

1. *Bodoia RD, Kinyoun JL, Qingli L, Bunt-Milam AH:* Aspergillus necrotizing retinitis: a clinico-pathologic study and review. Retina 9: 226-231, 1989
2. *Carney MD, Combs JL, Waschler W:* Cryptococcal choroiditis. Retina 10: 27-32, 1990
3. *Culbertson WW:* Infections of the retina in AIDS. Int Ophthalmol Clin 29: 108-118, 1989
4. *Davis JL, Nussenblatt RB, Bachmann DM, et al.:* Endogenous bacterial retinitis in AIDS. Am J Ophthalmol 107: 613-623, 1989
5. *Fabricius E-M:* Augenmanifestationen bei HIV-Infektionen. Bücherei des Augenarztes, Vol. 129, Enke, Stuttgart, pp. 49-134, 1992
6. *Forster DJ, Dugel PU, Frangieh GT, Liggett PE, Rao NA*: Rapidly progressive outer retinal necrosis in the acquired immunodeficiency syndrome. Am J Ophthalmol. 110: 341,1990
7. *Freeman WR, Gross JG, Labelle J, et al.:* Pneumocystis carinii choroidopathy. Arch Ophthalmol 107: 863-867, 1989
8. *Levy JH, Liss RA, Maguire AM:* Neurosyphilis and ocular syphilis in patients with concurrent human immunodeficiency virus infection. Retina 9: 175-180, 1989
9. *Qavi HB, Green MT, SeGall GK, Font RL:* Demonstration of HIV-1 and HHV-6 in AIDS-associated retinitis. Curr Eye Res 8: 379-387, 1989
10. *Rehder JR, Burnier M, Pavesio CE, et al.:* Acute unilateral toxoplasmic iridocyclitis in an AIDS-patient. Am J Ophthalmol 106: 740-741, 1988

3.27 Acute retinal necrosis

Etiology:

- HSV Type 1 and 2, VZV (CMV?)
- Most patients affected by acute retinal necrosis are immunocompetent
- The course of development, however, is similar to that of:
  - AIDS patients (however, CMV-retinitis is much more common)
  - Immunosuppressed patients
  - Newborn children (HSV-2) (probably intrauterine infection)
- Usually HSV retinitis in younger patients and VZV in older ones
- Genetic predisposition is possible: HLA-DQw7 has been found in 55% (vs. 19% in controls)

General involvement:

- Ophthalmic zoster or zoster dermatitis may precede the appearance of the retinal necrosis syndrome by weeks or years
- Involvement of the contralateral eye may develop later
- In immunosuppressed patients, the syndrome is a sign of possible other opportunistic infections

Ocular involvement:

- Usually begins with an anterior chamber reaction
- White, confluent areas of necrosis begin peripherally or (rarely) centrally
- All layers of the retina are affected
- Occlusive vasculitis, predominantly of the arteries
- Hemorrhage is present but markedly less than in CMV retinitis
- Usually a pronounced vitreous reaction
- Often optic nerve swelling
- Pigmentation of the necrosis areas within weeks; tractive detachment of the retina is caused by vitreous strands in 75% if no acyclovir therapy is given

- Recurrences are possible in previously unaffected retinal areas
- Bilateral in 35%
- Clinical differentiation between the various HSV types and VZV is still not possible; however, there are indications that retinitis induced by type 2 HSV may sometimes begin at the posterior pole and spread out peripherally

Diagnosis:

- Definition based solely on clinical appearance and course
  - Diagnostic criteria (1):
    1. One or more foci of retinal necrosis with discrete borders located in the peripheral retina
    2. Rapid progression of disease without antiviral therapy
    3. Circumferential spread of disease
    4. Evidence of occlusive vasculopathy with arteriolar involvement
    5. Prominent inflammatory reaction in the vitreous and anterior chamber
    6. Not required characteristics: optic neuropathy or atrophy, scleritis, pain
    7. If not all of these criteria are seen, the term 'necrotizing herpetic retinopathy' should be used.
- History of prior zoster infections
- Clinical picture:
  - Typical signs of retinitis
  - Differential diagnosis with regard to other forms of retinitis may not be possible
- Laboratory tests:
  - Virus isolation:
    - From vitreous or anterior chamber puncture specimens
      - Strongest confirmation
      - Absence of the antigen does not contradict the possibility of active infection
  - Antibody demonstration:
    - Individual tests yield little information; successive checks of vitreous puncture specimens give good results

- Demonstration of the viral genome:
  - with in-situ hybridization
  - with PCR
- Retinal biopsy:
  - Can be very hazardous
  - May permit differential diagnosis from other forms of retinitis through the use of other methods (immunohistochemical virus demonstration, in-vitro hybridization, PCR)

Remarks:
Our knowledge concerning the clinical course of the various forms of retinitis is growing rapidly, due above all to experience with AIDS-infected patients. The previous restriction of the designation 'Acute Retinal Necrosis' to patients who show no immunologic defects appears only partially appropriate and has not been included in the criteria of the American Uveitis Society, since these patients display no other opportunistic infections and thus have a different mortality rate than immunocompromised patients. On the other hand, the frequent history of zoster infections shows that the antiviral immune system may have defects which have previously received practically no study.

Literature:

1. *Holland, GN and the Executive Commitee of the American Uveitis Society:* Standard diagnostic criteria for the acute retinal necrosis syndrome. Am J Ophthalmol 117: 663-667,1994
2. *Duker JS, Fischer DH:* Herpes virus retinitis. Curr Opin Infect Dis 3: 555-558, 1990
3. *Fabricius E-M:* Augenmanifestationen bei HIV-Infektionen. Bücherei des Augenarztes, Vol. 129, Enke, Stuttgart, pp. 49-134, 1992
4. *Fisher JP, Lewis ML, Blumenkranz M et al.:* The acute retinal necrosis syndrome. Part 1: Clinical manifestations. Ophthalmology 89: 1309-1316, 1982
5. *Reynolds JD, Griebel M, Mallory S, Steele R:* Congenital herpes simplex retinitis. Am J Ophthalmol 102: 33-36, 1986

6. *Zierhut M, Thiel HJ, Weidle EG, Vallbracht A:* Akute nekrotisierende Retinitis nach Varizella-Zoster-Virus-Infektion. Klin Mbl Augenheilk 194: 52–58, 1989

3.28 Cytomegalovirus retinitis

Etiology:

- Cytomegalovirus infection of the retina
- Especially in patients with:
  - Defective T-cell system
  - AIDS (15–40% of AIDS patients)
  - Congenital CMV infection in newborn children (cytoplasmic inclusion disease)
  - After bone marrow transplantation
  - After kidney transplantation
  - Also possible in 'acute retinal necrosis syndrome' in apparently immunocompetent patients

General involvement:

Infection of newborn children:

- The most common intrauterine infection (ca. 1% of all live births)
- 5–10% of CMV-infected newborn children develop cytoplasmic inclusion disease with lesions of the reticuloendothelial system and the CNS
- 90–95% remain asymptomatic, develop psychomotor dysfunction or have impaired hearing

CMV infection in recipients of bone marrow or other transplants:

- Active CMV infection in 50–100% of the patients
- Reactivation during immunosuppressive therapy or transmission to seronegative recipients via seropositive tissue or blood
- Pneumonia, hepatitis, colitis, nephritis

CMV infection in AIDS:

- Cf. Chap. 3.26

CMV infection in immunocompetent patients:

- Fever, atypical lymphocytosis, abnormal liver function tests

Ocular involvement:

Three types of retinitis are distinguishable; however, they can appear simultaneously in the same eye:

- Hemorrhagic type:
  - Classic type
  - Necrotizing retinitis with extensive intraretinal bleeding
  - Usually at the posterior pole
- 'Bush fire' type:
  - Retinitis spreads like a bush fire due to cell-to-cell infection
  - Sharply defined yellowish-white margin, with atrophic scars behind it
  - Development of vitreo-chorioretinal adhesions with rhegmatogenous retinal detachment
- Granular type:
  - Especially in peripheral CMV and after treatment with Ganciclovir
  - Transition to the other two forms is possible
- Optic nerve involvement:
  - Small hemorrhages at the yellowish-white optic nerve
  - Possible transition to a neuroretinitis with massive deterioration of visual acuity
- Vasculitis:
  - Usually with perivenous sheathing, also in areas distant from the focus of retinitis
  - Arterial sheathing appears less common
- Changes in the corneal endothelium:
  - May occur as endotheliitis
  - The endothelium of AIDS patients may display either small, dark, round, mobile structures (lymphocytes?) or large, light-colored, spindle-shaped, stationary structures (macrophages?)
- Chorioretinitis:

- In cytoplasmic inclusion disease
- With optic nerve atrophy and cataract

Diagnosis:

- History and clinical picture
- Laboratory tests:
  - Virus isolation:
    - In vitreous or anterior chamber puncture specimens
      - This is the most definitive confirmation, but may take weeks
      - Detection of 'early nuclear antigen' by immunofluorescence as a marker of active infection
      - Absence of the antigen, however, does not exclude active infection

  - Antibody demonstration:
    - Is of little help
    - However, elevated IgM can be a sign of primary infection or reactivation
  - Demonstration of the viral genome
    - with PCR
    - with in-situ hybridization
- Retinal biopsy:
  - May be very hazardous
  - Histologically, 'owl-eye' inclusion bodies are found
  - May permit differential diagnostic exclusion of other forms of retinitis through the use of other methods (immunohistochemical virus demonstration, in-vitro hybridization)

Remarks:

CMV-retinitis in non-HIV positive patients seems to be less aggressive and more easily controllable

Literature:

1. *Hennis HL, Scott AA, Apple DJ:* Cytomegalovirus Retinitis. Surv Ophthalmol 34: 193–203. 1989

2. *Severin M, Hartmann C:* Endothelial alterations in AIDS with cytomegalovirus infection. Ophthalmologica, Basel 196: 7-10, 1988
3. *Wyhinny GJ, Apple DJ, Guastella FR, Vygantas CM:* Adult cytomegalic inclusion retinitis. Am J Ophthalmol 76: 773-781, 1973

E) Microorganism-induced uveitis

3.29 Herpes simplex uveitis

Etiology:
- Herpes simplex virus Type 1 (ocular-oral type) (HSV-1) and herpes simplex virus Type 2 (genital type) (HSV-2)
- Primary infection is followed by viral persistence in the corresponding ganglia (in the eye: the trigeminal ganglion)
- Reactivation occurs due to diverse stimuli (fever, steroids, menstruation, stress)
- The pathogenetic mechanism of HSV disease is traceable partly to a direct cytotoxic effect and partly to the immune system's subsequent defense reaction
- Recurrence is characteristic of HSV diseases
- Infection rate in the population is high; up to 80% for HSV-1 in Germany (from the 14th year of life on), lower for HSV-2

General involvement:
- Primary infection with HSV-1:
  - Subclinical development in 99%
  - Gingivostomatitis
  - Inoculation herpes (herpes whitlows on fingers sucked by children)
  - Varicelliform herpetic pustulosis
  - Meningoencephalitis
- Primary infection with HSV-2:
  - In newborn children:

    - Infection of the parietal channels
    - Viremia leading to:
    - Necrotic foci in the liver, spleen, adrenal glands, kidney, brain, lung, intestinal tract and skin
    - Icterus, lethargy, vomiting, dyspnea, cyanosis, swollen liver
    - Usually fatal
    - Incidence: 1:3,500 live births
  - Herpes genitalis in adults and teenagers
- Reactivation of HSV-1:
  - Herpes labialis (lips, mouth, but also on the external genitals and other areas of the skin)
  - Occasionally with regional lymphadenopathy
  - Repeated infection of the same skin area is usual

Ocular involvement:

- Primary infection with HSV-1:
  - Incubation period: 3-9 days
  - Fever, malaise, pre-auricular lymph node swelling
  - Eyelid infection, conjunctivitis, mild keratitis
  - Mild iritis (unilateral in 95%)
  - Very benign development without scarring
  - Infection usually between the 6th month and 5th year of life for HSV-1 and the 16th and 25th year of life for HSV-2
- Primary infection with HSV-2:
  - Ocular involvement in 82%
  - Mainly in newborn children
- Reactivation of HSV-1:
  - Blepharitis
  - Dendritic keratitis
  - Diverse forms of interstitial keratitis (including disciform keratitis)
  - Endotheliitis
  - Iritis, often as keratouveitis with trabeculitis:
    - Reduced corneal sensitivity if the cornea is involved

    - Secondary glaucoma
    - Rapid formation of synechiae
    - Focal defect of the pigment epithelium of the iris
    - Spontaneous anterior chamber hemorrhages
  - Optic nerve neuritis, papillitis
  - Retinitis, retinochoroiditis:
    - White, confluent spots originating peripherally
    - Intraretinal bleeding and exudation
    - Usually a pronounced vitreous reaction
    - Exudative retinal detachment
    - Papillitis
    - Often bilateral
    - Sometimes also a discrete picture
    - The immune system is usually intact in the discrete form
    - Massive reaction:
      - In patients with weakened immune responses, such as after bone marrow or kidney transplantation, under cytostatic therapy for malignancy or in newborn children whose immune system is not yet fully developed
      - In combination with acute retinal necrosis in clinically otherwise healthy patients (cf. Chap. 3.27)
      - Occasionally develops together with other signs of HSV reactivation (meningoencephalitis), even in otherwise healthy persons
- Reactivation of HSV-2:
  - In contrast to HSV-1:
  - Iritis; the course is probably much more severe
  - Retinitis:
    - More commonly induced in newborn children by HSV-2
    - The role of HSV-2 in adults is not yet clear

Diagnosis:
- History:
  - Possible indications of recurrent keratitis or
  - Immunosuppression (retinitis, panuveitis)

- Clinical picture: keratouveitis prompts early suspicion of HSV; however, the symptoms may be uncharacteristic (no corneal involvement)
- Laboratory tests: direct demonstration of pathogens:
  - Possible in aqueous or vitreous puncture specimens
  - Negative results do not eliminate HSV, since HSV spreads from cell to cell
  - Through in-vitro hybridization: pathogens may be found in retinal biopsy specimens

Remarks:

HSV-iritis represents a major diagnostic problem. If recurrent iritis responds poorly to steroids and rapidly leads to secondary glaucoma, repeated HSV-tests should be carried out in the aqueous humor.

Literature:

1. *Chang TS, Brewer LV, Hooper PL:* Primary herpes simplex iridocyclitis with iris atrophy. Arch Ophthalmol 111: 25-26, 1993
2. *Colin J, Renard G, Chastel C:* Ocular infection due to herpex simplex virus type 2. In: Immunology and Immunopathology of the Eye. Silverstein AM, O'Connor GR (Editors), Masson, New York, pp. 279-281, 1979
3. *Sundmacher R:* A clinico-virologic classification of herpetic anterior segment disease with special reference to intraocular herpes. In: Herpetische Augenerkrankungen, Sundmacher R (Editor), Bergmann, Munich, pp. 203-208, 1981
4. *Thygeson P, Ostler HB:* Zoster and herpes simplex virus uveitis: a comparison. In: Immunology and Immunopathology of the Eye. Silverstein AM, O'Connor GR (Editors), Masson, New York, pp. 230-240, 1979

3.30 Varicella zoster uveitis

Etiology:

- Infection with VZV
- Causes varicella in children
- Persists in the involved ganglion (in the eye: the trigeminal ganglion)
- Reactivation for various reasons (cytostatic therapy, in AIDS, in tumors), but the cause is often unknown
- Gains access to the eye via the 1st branch of the trigeminal nerve
- Involvement of the tip of the nose (nasociliary nerve) is a sign of impending ocular involvement

General involvement:

- Fever, general malaise
- Intense regional pain around the afflicted nerve
- Maculopapular skin lesions in the region after 1–2 days
- Cerebral arteriitis with neurologic defects

Ocular involvement:

- Ocular involvement in 50–70% of patients with affected trigeminus
- Conjunctivitis
- Keratitis (including a dendritic, a disciform and a neurotrophic form)
- Episcleritis, scleritis (a rare late manifestation)
- Optic nerve neuritis
- Anterior uveitis with keratitis (30%):
  - Damage to the iris sphincter is characteristic
  - Segmental iris atrophy
  - Secondary glaucoma (10%)
- Retinitis:
  - On rare occasions simultaneous with zoster ophthalmicus
  - Occasionally subsequent to zoster ophthalmicus or zoster dermatitis

- In this case it may involve the other eye as well
- Clinical picture as in acute retinal necrosis (cf. Chap. 3.27)

Diagnosis:

- The case history and clinical picture are typical in zoster ophthalmicus but not in VZV retinitis
- Laboratory tests: direct demonstration of pathogens:
  - In the anterior chamber or vitreous puncture specimen if the overall picture is unclear (i.e. usually in retinitis), via culture or PCR techniques
  - VZV can be demonstrated in retinal biopsies via in-vitro hybridization
- Identification of the cause:
  - Search for possible underlying malignancies
  - HIV test (esp. in younger patients)

Remarks:

Younger patients with zoster ophthalmicus remain HIV-suspects until proven otherwise, i.e. even a negative HIV test should be repeated after some time. Post-traumatic ophthalmic zoster keratitis can be the first sign of a HIV infection (cf. Chap. 3.26).

Literature:

1. *Cobo M, Foulks GN, Liesegang T, et al.:* Observations on the natural history of herpes zoster ophthalmicus. Curr Eye Res 6: 195-199, 1987
2. *Sundmacher R:* Die fokale Iritis durch Herpes simplex- und Varizella-Zoster-Virus. Ber Dtsch Ophthalmol Ges 78: 73-76, 1981
3. *Womack LW, Liesegang ThJ:* Complications of Herpes Zoster ophthalmicus. Arch Ophthalmol 101: 42-45, 1983

3.31 Epstein-Barr virus uveitis

Etiology:

- There is as yet no unequivocal proof of an EBV-caused uveitis or retinitis
- In all cases reported to date there have been serologic indications of acute EBV infection

General involvement:

- Primary EBV infection in childhood almost always has an asymptomatic course
- Mononucleosis can develop during reactivation
- Chronic illness in combination with persisting EBV and an inadequate immune system can lead to severe diseases such as Burkitt's lymphoma or nasopharyngeal carcinoma

Ocular involvement:

- Conjunctivitis, usually follicular, in combination with acute EBV infection (mononucleosis)
- Keratitis in an epithelial and a stromal form
- Sjögren's syndrome
- Chronic, usually bilateral iridocyclitis in combination with chronic EBV infections
- Multifocal choroiditis (cf. Chap. 3.24)

Diagnosis:

- Clinical picture:
  - Leads to a presumed diagnosis only in the case of multifocal choroiditis
- Laboratory tests:
  - Demonstration of antibodies:
    - Possible against various EBV antigens
    - VCA = virus-capsid-antigen (IgG and IgM)
    - EA = early antigen (IgG and IgM)
    - EBNA = Epstein-Barr nuclear antigen

- An acute or persisting infection is characterized by elevated EA-antibodies and VCA-IgM antibodies (beginning ca. 4–5 weeks after exposure)
- These antibodies remain elevated only 6–12 months after the onset of the disease, whereas VCA-IgG and EBNA remain permanently demonstrable

Remarks:

The role of EBV as a pathogen in uveitis remains highly controversial. Due to the high rate of contamination in the population, positive serologic results are to be treated with great caution.

Literature:

1. *Spaide RF, Sugin S, Yannuzzi LA, DeRosa JT:* Epstein-Barr virus antibodies in multifocal choroiditis and panuveitis. Am J Ophthalmol 112: 410–413, 1991
2. *Tidemann JS:* Epstein-Barr viral antibodies in multifocal choroiditis and panuveitis. Am J Ophthalmol 103: 659–663, 1987
3. *Wong KW, D'Amico DJ, Hedges TR et al.:* Ocular involvement associated with chronic Epstein-Barr virus disease. Arch Ophthalmol 105: 788–792, 1987

3.32 Rubella

Etiology:

- Congenital infection by the rubella virus
- Particularly dangerous in the first 2 months of pregnancy
- Lack of immunity to rubella in 15% of women of childbearing age

General involvement:

- Rubella embryopathy
- Often stillbirth or premature birth; otherwise deafness, CNS deficiencies or cardiac defects

- Acquired rubella infection:
  - Influenza-like infection with erythema
  - Occasionally subclinical

Ocular involvement:
- Cataract
- Glaucoma
- Microphthalmia
- Nystagmus, strabismus
- Chorioretinitis:
  - Usually subsides before birth
  - Hyper- and hypopigmented areas of scars
  - Subretinal neovascularization membranes
  - Vitreous tractions with retinal detachment

Diagnosis:
- History:
  - Possible rubella infection during pregnancy
- Laboratory tests: demonstration of antibodies
  - An elevation of IgM antibodies indicates that an infection ran its course a short time ago

Literature:

1. *Deutman AF, Grizzard WS:* Rubella retinopathy and subretinal neovascularization. Am J Ophthalmol 85: 82-87, 1978
2. *Frank KE, Purnell EW:* Subretinal neovascularization following rubella retinopathy. Am J Ophthalmol 86: 462-466, 1978
3. *Hertzberg R:* Twenty-five year follow-up of ocular defects in congenital rubella. Am J Ophthalmol 66: 269-271, 1968

3.33 Subacute sclerosing panencephalitis

Etiology:
- Slow-virus infection (measles?)
- Typically months or years after an early measles infection

- Histopathology: infiltration of lymphocytes and monocytes, especially in the small arteries and veins
- Children and teenagers are affected (60–90% male)
- Progressive development, invariably fatal

General involvement:

- Onset with personality changes
- Impaired coordination

Ocular involvement:

- Nystagmus, eye muscle pareses
- Optic nerve atrophy
- Retinitis:
  - Usually at the posterior pole
  - Retinal hemorrhage
  - No vitreous reaction

Diagnosis:

- History: look for measles
- Laboratory tests:
  - Direct demonstration of measles:
    - Sometimes possible in tissue
    - The relevance is not clear
  - Demonstration of antibodies:
    - Positive results for anti-measles antibodies in serum and spinal fluid can be regarded as confirmation of the diagnosis

Literature:

1. *Deutman AF, Scheffer CT, Binkhorst PG:* Subacute sclerosing panencephalitis. Ophthalmologica 173: 430–431, 1976
2. *Kovacs B, Vastag O:* Fluoroangiographic picture of the acute stage of the retinal lesion in subacute sclerosing panencephalitis. Ophthalmologica 177: 264–269, 1978

3. *Robb RM, Watters GV:* Ophthalmic manifestation of subacute sclerosing panencephalitis. Arch Ophthalmol 83: 425–435, 1970

3.34 Rift Valley fever

Etiology:

- Infection by an RNA virus of the arbovirus group
- Disease of domestic animals (sheep, cattle)
- Transmission to humans by biting insects
- Endemic to southern Africa, Egypt, and the Sudan

General involvement:

- 3- to 7-day incubation period
- Prodromal stage with biphasic febrile course (subsiding after the 2nd or 3rd day of illness)
- Retro-orbital pain, photophobia
- Arthralgias
- Rarely encephalitis, hepatitis

Ocular involvement:

- Usually 1–3 weeks after onset of illness
- Retinitis with vasculitis:
  - Cotton-wool spots
  - Intraretinal bleeding
  - Retinal edema with macular involvement
  - Possible epiretinal fibrosis with tractive retinal detachment

Diagnosis:

- History: previous trips to countries with endemic Rift Valley fever
- Laboratory tests:
  - Demonstration of antibodies:
    - Elevated specific antibodies (CFR, hemagglutination inhibition test)

- Direct demonstration of pathogens:
  - Possible in the serum

Literature:

1. *Conrads H, Wittwer K, Bichmann W:* Rift-Valley-Fieber: Ungewöhnlicher Verlauf einer tropischen Erkrankung mit Augenbeteiligung. Klin Mbl Augenheilk 185: 397–399, 1984
2. *Deutmann AF, Klomp HJ:* Rift valley fever retinitis. Am J Ophthalmol 92: 38–42, 1981
3. *Siam AL, Meegan JM, Gharbawi KF:* Rift valley fever ocular manifestations: observations during the 1977 epidemic in Egypt. Br J Ophthalmol 64: 366–374, 1980

3.35 Rocky Mountain spotted fever

Etiology:

- Infection with Rickettsia rickettsii
- Transmitted by ticks
- Histology: necrosis of the interna and media of blood vessels, followed by occlusion
- The disease occurs in North, Central and South America

General involvement:

- First clinical symptoms 1–2 weeks after tick bite
- Prodromal stage: headache, myalgia
- Exanthema on the 4th day of illness
  - Characterized by scattered areas of pink rash 1–4 mm in diameter, beginning at the extremities and spreading rapidly centrally
- Usually heals without defects
- Rarely: liver and kidney involvement

Ocular involvement:

- Spotty conjunctival bleeding
- Conjunctivitis

- Iridocyclitis
- Retinitis:
  - Retinal bleeding
  - Cotton-wool spots
  - Occlusion of retinal vessels
- Optic disc edema

Diagnosis:
- History:
  - Previous stays in endemic areas
  - Tick bites, but these are often forgotten
- Laboratory tests: demonstration of antibodies:
  - From the 7th to 10th day of illness on (agglutinating antibodies in the Weil-Felix test)
  - In the complement fixation reaction after 10 to 14 days
  - Increased sensitivity of immunofluorescence
  - Antibody demonstration only for a few weeks

Literature:

1. *Presley GD:* Fundus changes in Rocky Mountain spotted fever. Am J Ophthalmol 67: 263-267, 1969
2. *Smith TW, Buron TC:* The retinal manifestations of Rocky Mountain Spotted Fever. Am J Ophthalmol 84: 259-262, 1977
3. *Sulewski ME, Green WR:* Ocular histopathologic features of a presumed case of Rocky Mountain Spotted Fever. Retina 6: 125-130, 1986

3.36 Trypanosomiasis

Etiology:
- Infection by Trypanosoma gambiense (south of the Sahara, west of the Rift Valley), Trypanosoma brucei rhodesiense (Ethiopia to Botswana) or Trypanosoma cruzi (Central and South America)

- Hemoflagellates, transmitted by insect bites
- Organs are affected due to parasitemia
- Histopathology: vasculitis with infiltration by plasma cells and polymorphonuclear leucocytes
- T. gambiense and T. rhodesiense induce sleeping sickness
- T. cruzi induces Chagas' disease
- Ocular involvement induced by trypanosomiasis is rare

General involvement:

- African sleeping disease:
  - Primary lesion with lymphadenopathy
  - Prodromal complaints: headache, fever
  - Splenomegaly
  - CNS and cardiac involvement
  - Demyelinating panencephalitis
  - Slow progression over years
- American Chagas' disease:
  - the primary lesion is usually at the point of transition from skin to mucosa
  - Lymphadenopathy, hepatosplenomegaly
  - Cardiac involvement (10%) may be fatal

Ocular involvement:

- Recurrent lid edema
- Eyelid chagoma (inflammatory-edematous primary focus at the portal of entry of T. cruzi)
- Dacryocystitis (T. cruzi)
- Conjunctival chemosis
- Diffuse interstitial keratitis
- Iridocyclitis, possibly granulomatous
- Retinitis:
  - Intraretinal bleeding
  - Granulomatous retinal infiltrate
  - Vasculitis
- Optic neuritis with optic nerve atrophy

Diagnosis:

- History: travel in endemic areas
- Laboratory tests: Direct demonstration of pathogens:
  - Occasionally possible in smear preparations (blood, spinal fluid, lymph-node tissue)
  - Demonstration of antibodies

Literature:

1. *Huismans H:* Tierische Parasiten des menschlichen Auges. Bücherei des Augenarztes Vol. 80, Enke, Stuttgart, 1979, pp. 36–46

3.37 Amebiasis

Etiology:

- Infection by Entamoeba histolytica or Acanthamoebae
- Transmitted by contaminated water or food or as a consequence of poor contact-lens hygiene
- Ocular involvement is rare

General involvement:

- Chronic elimination after infection
- Gastrointestinal problems
- Rarely, liver abscesses and peritonitis

Ocular involvement:

- Entamoeba histolytica:
  - Intermediate uveitis
  - Choroiditis
    - Subretinal, white, granulomatous or plaque-like exudative lesion (cyst)
    - Usually located in the macula
    - Frequent distortion of the retinal pigment epithelium
  - Optic neuritis
  - Pseudotumor

- Acanthamoebae:
  - Keratitis (by direct corneal infection)
  - Keratouveitis (transmitted)
  - Chorioretinitis as in E. histolytica

Diagnosis:

- History: Acanthamoebae in contact-lens wearers
- Clinical picture: infection with Acanthamoebae is extremely painful
- Laboratory tests:
  - Direct demonstration of pathogens:
    - E. histolytica: analysis of stool samples and possibly of the cerebrospinal fluid in case of CNS involvement; abscess puncture specimens
    - Acanthamoebae: immunofluorescent analysis of corneal ulcus and demonstration in special cultures (Chalkofluor)
  - Antibody demonstration:
    - Only in case of extraintestinal infection by E. histolytica

Literature:

1. *Harris D, Birch CL:* Bilateral uveitis associated with gastrointestinal Entamoeba-histolytica infection. Am J Ophthalmol 50: 496-500, 1960
2. *Jones DB, Visvesvara GS, Robinson NM:* Acanthamoeba polyphaga keratitis and Acanthamoeba uveitis associated with fatal meningoencephalitis. Trans Ophthalmol Soc UK 95: 221-232, 1975
3. *King RE, Praeger DL, Hallett JW:* Amebic choroiditis. Arch Ophthalmol 72: 16-22, 1964

3.38 Cysticercosis

Etiology:

- Immune reaction to dead larvae (Cystercicus cellulosae) of Taenia solium

- After ingestion, the eggs mature and larvae penetrate the mucosa, leading to organ manifestations
- Found in Eastern Europe, Central and South America, Africa, Southeast Asia

General involvement:
- Development of cysts or:
- Diverse organ manifestations, e.g.:
- CNS involvement (40%)
- Skin (6 %)
- In general, systemic involvement is often unobtrusive

Ocular involvement:
- Ptosis
- Subconjunctival, hemispheric, cystic, contact-sensitive tumor, often in the inferior conjunctival fornix
- Iritis, iridocyclitis
- Chorioretinitis:
  - Subretinal cyst
  - Can intrude into the vitreous, where it moves around freely
- Optic nerve neuritis, optic disc atrophy
- Impaired motility
- Pseudotumor of the orbit

Diagnosis:
- History: Check foreign travel
- Clinical picture: subretinal cysts are often very characteristic
- Laboratory tests:
  - Direct demonstration of pathogens:
    - Worm eggs in the stool (only rarely found)
  - Demonstration of antibodies:
    - The indirect hemagglutination inhibition test is 80% specific because of the presence of cross-reactions
    - Eosinophilia: in blood and anterior chamber puncture specimens

Literature:

1. *Kruger-Leite E, Jalkh AE, Quiroz H, Schepens ChL:* Intraocular cysticercosis. Am J Ophthalmol 99: 252–257, 1985
2. *Messner KH, Kammerer WS:* Intraocular cysticercosis. Arch Ophthalmol 97: 1103–1105, 1979
3. *Wessing A, Meyer-Schwickerath G:* Intraokularer Zystizerkus und Behandlung mit dem 'vitreous suction cutter' (VISC). Klin Mbl Augenheilk 165: 865–867, 1974

3.39 Echinococcosis

Etiology:

- Reaction to larvae of E. granulosus or E. multilocularis
- After uptake of the eggs, the larvae pass into the liver via the gastric mucosa and the portal vein, and are distributed thereafter hematogenously
- Primarily found in sheep-breeding countries
- Prognosis: usually fatal unless surgically removed

General involvement:

- Lung cysts (60%)
- Liver cysts (40%)
- CNS involvement
- Decade-long development is typical

Ocular involvement:

- Tautly elastic eyelid tumor
- Conjunctival chemosis
- Impaired motility
- Orbital tumor
- Chorioretinitis:
  - Focal
  - Yellowish, subretinal infiltrate
  - Development of intraocular cysts
  - Pronounced anterior chamber reaction is possible

Diagnosis:

- Laboratory tests: Demonstration of antibodies:
  - Possibly present in the blood, but cross-reactions are frequent
  - Eosinophilia (not always present)
- Sonography: demonstration of cysts
- X-ray: bone erosions when perforation of the orbital roof is imminent; demonstration of calcification

Literature:

1. *Bernsmeier H:* Subretinaler Echinokokkus. Klin Mbl Augenheilk 177: 85-87, 1980
2. *Huismans H:* Tierische Parasiten des menschlichen Auges. Bücherei des Augenarztes Vol. 80, Enke, Stuttgart, 1979, pp. 75-84
3. *Williams DF, Williams GA, Caya JG, et al.:* Intraocular Echinococcus multilocularis. Arch Ophthalmol 105: 1106-1109, 1987

3.40 Ophthalmomyiasis

Etiology:

- Immunologic reaction to larvae of Diptera (two-winged insects), usually from the sub-group Cyclorrhapha
- The larvae are usually deposited on the eyelids, from where they can migrate into the eye
- Found ubiquitously, but most frequently in rural areas of the Mediterranean, Africa and Russia
- Most often affected are children, ill persons and alcoholics; contact with animals and poor hygiene are predisposing factors
- The larvae mature in the nasal mucosa of the primary host (cattle, horses, sheep)
- Ophthalmomyiasis is probably caused by mistakes in scent and vision: dark eyes are mistaken for the dark cavities of the nostrils!

General involvement:
- None

Ocular involvement:
- Ophthalmomyiasis externa:
  - Conjunctivitis is the most frequent form, prognosis is good
  - Orbital myiasis with painful exophthalmos and development of edema, dacryocystitis
- Ophthalmomyiasis interna:
  - Luxation of the lens
  - Iridocyclitis (occasionally with hypopyon)
  - Panuveitis
  - Striate changes of the retinal pigment epithelium due to subretinal migration of the larvae; subretinal or intravitreal cysts
  - Migration into the optic nerve is possible
  - Occasional retinal detachment
  - Or: the larvae can remain in the eye with no flare
  - Transmitted especially by flies of the hypoderma group
  - The ocular prognosis is very poor

Diagnosis:
- History: Contact with flies is usually reported
- Clinical picture: The larva is sometimes seen
- Determination of larvae should always be undertaken

Remarks:
The disease is normally unusual in central Europe and the United States, but tourism has increased its incidence.

Literature:

1. *Cameron JA, Shoukrey NM, Al-Garni AA:* Conjunctival ophthalmomyiasis caused by the sheep nasal botfly (Oestrus ovis). Am J Ophthalmol 112: 331–334, 1991
2. *Fitzgerald CR, Rubin ML:* Intraocular parasite destroyed by photocoagulation. Arch Ophthalmol 91: 162–164, 1974

3. *Slusher MM, Holland WD, Weaver RG, Tyler ME:* Ophthalmomyiasis interna posterior, subretinal tracks and intraocular larvae. Arch Ophthalmol 97: 885-887, 1979

3.41 Giardiasis

Etiology:

- Reaction to the protozoon Giardia lamblia
- Infection by contaminated food or drinking water
- Mobile form (trophozoite) or cystic form
- Multiplies in the intestines

General involvement:

- Stomach cramps, diarrhea, constipation, weight loss
- Headache, nervousness, emotional instability

Ocular involvement:

- Recurrent eyelid edema
- Episcleritis
- Iridocyclitis
- Chorioiditis
- Retinal hemorrhages
- Vasculitis
- Papillitis

Diagnosis:

- History: history of travel
- Laboratory tests: direct demonstration of pathogens:
  - in the stool (cysts); only occasionally successful; increased elimination after administration of magnesium sulfate
- Biopsy: intestinal mucosa

Literature:

1. *Knox DL, King J Jr:* Retinal arteritis, iridocyclitis, and giardiasis. Ophthalmology 89: 1303-1308. 1982

2. *Webster BH:* Human infection with Giardia lamblia. An analysis of 32 cases. Am J Dig Dis (New Series) 3: 64–71, 1958

3.42 Onchocerciasis

Etiology:

- Immunologic reaction to disintegrating microfilariae of Onchocerca volvulus and their metabolic products
- Most common intraocular inflammation (more than 50 million humans afflicted, with blindness in 10%)
- Found from western to central Africa, in Central America, with scattered cases in northern South America and on the Arabian peninsula

General involvement:

- Skin nodules (adult worm), especially on the head and trunk
- Chronic dermatosis with pruritus due to migration of the microfilariae ('lizard skin', irregular pigmentation)

Ocular involvement:

- Painfully swollen eyelids, blepharospasm
- Conjunctivitis (onset of migration), phlyctenoid efflorescences, later deposition of gray-brown pigment
- Keratitis (the major complication, the only ocular involvement in 45%): onset with wave-like opacification in the upper stroma, especially in the area of the limbus; later pterygium-like limbal conjunctival proliferation and sclerosing keratitis
- Iridocyclitis
  - Often with secondary glaucoma and pseudohypopyon (dead microfilariae)
- Chorioretinitis:
  - May be exudative, leaving behind atrophic spots
  - Retinal hemorrhages
  - Macular degeneration
- Optic nerve neuritis, optic nerve atrophy

Diagnosis:

- History: history of travel
- Clinical picture:
  - If onchocerciasis is suspected, look for microfilariae: let the patient sit for several minutes in a dark room with his head between his knees, then examine the anterior chamber in the slit lamp
  - Skin changes: onchocercomas (demonstration of microfilariae)
- Laboratory tests:
  - Direct demonstration of parasites, e.g. in the skin and conjunctiva

Remarks:

The disease rarely presents difficulties in differential diagnosis; it is rare outside the third world, but should always be thought of in the corresponding patients, since Ivermectin is an effective means of treatment (cf. Vol. 2).

Literature:

1. *Bird AC, Anderson J, Fuglsang H:* Morphology of posterior segment lesions of the eye in patients with onchocerciasis. Br J Ophthalmol 60: 2-20, 1976
2. *Budden FH:* Ocular lesions of onchocerciasis. Br J Ophthalmol 46: 1-11, 1962
3. *Rothova A, Van der Lelij A, Stilma JS, et al.:* Ocular involvement in patients with onchocerciasis after repeated treatment with ivermectin. Am J Ophthalmol 110: 6-16, 1990

3.43 Ophthalmia nodosa

Etiology:

- A reaction to broken-off caterpillar hairs, which contain histamine-liberating substances
- Caterpillars can come into contact with the eye in various ways

General involvement:

- None

Ocular involvement:

- Granulomatous conjunctivitis when exclusively superficial
- Keratitis
- Iridocyclitis
  - Painful; followed by:
- Chorioretinal tracks:
  - These typically run from the anterior segment to the posterior pole
  - White nodules along the tracks
  - The start of migration can apparently be delayed for many years after contact with the hair

Diagnosis:

- Clinical picture

Literature:

1. *Cadera W, Pachtman MA, Fountain JA, et al.:* Ocular lesions caused by caterpillar hairs (ophthalmia nodosa). Can J Ophthalmol 19: 40–44, 1984
2. *Hered RW, Spaulding AG, Sanitato JJ, Wander AH:* Ophthalmia nodosa caused by tarantula hairs. Ophthalmology 95: 166–169, 1988
3. *Watson PG, Sevel D.:* Ophthalmia nodosa. Br J Ophthalmol 50: 209–217, 1966

3.44 Diffuse unilateral subacute neuroretinitis

Etiology:

- A reaction to nematodes, possibly to Baylisascaris procyonis (transmitted by raccoons) or Toxocara canis
- The disease has previously been described only in the USA and recently in Germany
- The prognosis is usually poor

General involvement:

- Occasional skin rash

Ocular involvement:

- Retinitis:
  - Scattered gray-white retinal lesions
  - Moderate or no vitreous reaction
  - Optic disc swelling, later optic nerve atrophy
  - Alterations of the pigment epithelium
  - Vascular constriction
  - The worm is located subretinally, sometimes in the vitreous

Diagnosis:

- Clinical picture:
  - With magnified ophthalmoscopy, a worm can be seen moving in the subretinal space
- Electrophysiology:
  - ERG clearly reduced
- Fluorescein angiography:
  - Early phase: no staining of the white spots
  - Late phase: staining of the spots, window defects
- Laboratory tests:
  - Pathogens have not yet been directly demonstrated
  - Antibody tests:
    - Until now, lowered anti-Toxocara antibody titers have been found occasionally
  - Occasional eosinophilia

Remarks:

The relevance of this picture for Europe is not yet known.

Literature:

1. *Gass JDM, Braunstein RA:* Further observations concerning the diffuse unilateral subacute neuroretinitis syndrome. Arch Ophthalmol 101: 1689–1697, 1983

2. *Kazacos KR, Vestre WA, Kazacos EA, Raymond LA:* Diffuse unilateral subacute neuroretinitis syndrome: A probable cause. Arch Ophthalmol 102: 967–968, 1984
3. *Kazacos KR, Raymond LA, Kazacos EA, Vestre WA:* The raccoon ascarid: A probable cause of human ocular larva migrans. Ophthalmology 92: 1735–1744, 1985

3.45 Candidiasis

Etiology:

- Infection with Candida
- Predisposing factors:
  - Immunosuppression (AIDS, malignancy)
  - Antibiotic therapy, steroid therapy
  - Diabetes mellitus
  - Intravenous drug use
  - Long-term intravenous therapy
- Ocular involvement usually combined with sepsis
- Most common cause of a fungal metastatic ocular inflammation

General involvement:

- Sepsis:
  - Relatively asymptomatic, or:
  - Fever, myalgia
  - Meningitis
  - Organ abscesses (lungs, brain)

Ocular involvement:

- Iridocyclitis with occasional hypopyon
- Chorioretinitis:
  - Whitish-yellow, fluffy spots of various size
  - Lead to densification of the overlying vitreous
  - Usually massive vitreous infiltration (depending on the patient's immune status)

- Vascular sheathing
- If the vitreous is infiltrated, there follows:

- Endophthalmitis:
  - Vitreous abscess
  - Anterior chamber reaction
- Gradual development of the ocular symptoms
- Usually bilateral
- Ocular involvement in 70% in Candida sepsis

Diagnosis:

- History: predisposing factors
- Laboratory tests:
  - Direct demonstration of pathogens
    - Blood cultures (often negative in drug addicts)
    - Aqueous and vitreous cultures
  - Microscopic demonstration:
    - In aqueous or vitreous puncture specimens: difficult, since often not sufficiently enriched
    - In culture

Remarks:

A large number of unknown cases can be assumed. A positive blood culture does not prove the existence of ocular Candida infection, since highly immunosuppressed or otherwise ill patients often display several opportunistic infections.

Literature:

1. *Aguilar GL, Blumenkrantz MS, Egbert PR, McCulley JP:* Candida endophthalmitis after intravenous drug abuse. Arch Ophthalmol 97: 96-100, 1979
2. *Brooks RG:* Prospective study of Candida endophthalmitis in hospitalized patients with candidemia. Arch Intern Med 149: 2226-2228, 1989
3. *Messerli J, Wegmann T, Speiser P:* Candida-Endophthalmitis bei Drogensüchtigen. Klin Mbl Augenheilk 184: 466-467, 1984

3.46 Endogenous mycotic endophthalmitis

Etiology:

- Metastatic
- Pathogens:
  - Candida (esp. in intravenous drug use or chronic intravenous therapy; 75–80% of all mycotic endophthalmitis (cf. Chap. 3.45)
  - Aspergillus fumigatus (in intravenous drug use, immunosuppression)
  - Geotrichum candidum
  - Cryptococcus neoformans (immunosuppression, lymphoma, AIDS)
  - Histoplasma capsulatum (immunosuppression, AIDS)
  - Sporotrichum schenckii (risk group: gardeners)
  - Blastomyces dermatidis (in systemic blastomycosis)
  - Mucor racemosus
  - Fusarium
- Predisposing factors:
  - Immunosuppression (malignant diseases, steroid treatment, antibody deficiencies, in newborn children)
  - Diabetes mellitus
  - Cardiac disease
  - Kidney failure
  - Postoperative period
  - Drug addiction

General involvement:

- Severe systemic or organic disease
  - Osteomyelitis
  - Lung abscess
  - Meningitis, cerebral abscess
- Occasional fever, muscle or joint pains as a sign of sepsis

Ocular involvement:

- Retinitis/choroiditis:
  - Fluffy, yellowish-white, round, choroidal or retinal spots
  - Often with hemorrhages
  - Spots become prominent
  - May invade the vitreous, causing development of:
- Endophthalmitis:
  - With additional iritis and
  - Massive anterior chamber flare, with hypopyon
- The development is usually gradual
- Little or no pain
- Candida (cf. Chap. 3.45)

Diagnosis:

- History:
  - Predisposing factors
- Clinical picture:
  - Search for spots; this is usually easy
- Laboratory tests:
  - Direct demonstration of pathogens:
    - Diagnostic vitrectomy
    - Blood cultures may be difficult

Remarks:

It can be assumed that the number of unknown cases in severely ill patients is very high.

Literature:

1. *Elliott JH, O'Day DM, Gutwow GS, et al.:* Mycotic endophthalmitis in drug abusers. Am J Ophthalmol 88: 66-72, 1979
2. *Font RL, Jakobiec FA:* Granulomatous necrotizing retinochoroiditis caused by Sporotrichum schenckii. Arch Ophthalmol 94: 1513-1519, 1976
3. *Lance SE, Friberg TR, Kowalski RP:* Aspergillus flavus en-

dophthalmitis and retinitis in an intravenous drug abuser. Ophthalmology 95: 947-949, 1988

3.47 Coccidioidomycosis

Etiology:

- Caused by the fungus Coccidioides immitis
- Ocular involvement follows hematogenous spread
- Histopathologically, granulomas are found near the vessels
- Outbreaks of the disease are confined for the most part to the area of contagion (North, Central and South America)
- USA: 100,000 cases a year

General involvement:

- Pulmonary involvement:
  - Asymptomatic (60%)
  - Infection of the respiratory tract (40%): mild course, with fever
- Erythema nodosum (5-10%)
- Fungemia (0.5%)
- Occasional CNS-involvement
- Risk of contagion seems independent of apparent predisposing factors
- The prognosis is good

Ocular involvement:

- Phlyctenular conjunctivitis
- Episcleritis, scleritis
- Iridocyclitis, usually mild
- Multifocal choroiditis:
  - Whitish-yellow granulomas, oval, slightly prominent
  - Characterized by few symptoms

Diagnosis:

- History: sojourns in contagious areas

- Laboratory tests:
  - Direct demonstration of pathogens
    - Sputum cultures
    - Blood cultures
  - Demonstration of antibodies:
    - From the 1st to 3rd week after infection
    - Persisting for 4-6 months

Literature:

1. *Blumenkranz MS, Stevens DA:* Endogenous coccidioidal endophthalmitis. Ophthalmology 87: 974-984, 1980
2. *Glasgow BJ, Brown HH, Foos RY:* Miliary retinitis in coccidioidomycosis. Am J Ophthalmol 104: 24-27, 1987
3. *Rodenbiker HT, Ganley JP, Galgiani JN, Axline StG:* Prevalence of chorioretinal scars associated with coccidioidomycosis. Arch Ophthalmol 99: 71-75, 1981

3.48 Cryptococcosis

Etiology:

- Infection by the yeast Cryptococcus neoformans
- Intake via the gastrointestinal tract, the respiratory tract or the skin
- Ocular involvement in combination with fungemia
- Histopathologically: granulomatous reaction
- Prevalent world-wide
- Probably a rare disease (USA: an estimated 300 cases per year)

General involvement:

- CNS involvement:
  - Meningitis, meningoencephalitis
  - Disorientation
  - Hydrocephalus
- Good prognosis if treated promptly

Ocular involvement:

- Cranial nerve pareses, nystagmus, optic disc swelling
- Iridocyclitis is rare
- Multifocal choroiditis/retinitis:
  - Multiple small foci
  - Hemorrhages
  - Vitreous reaction with tractive detachment is rare
- Ocular involvement in 40% with CNS involvement

Diagnosis:

- Direct demonstration of pathogens:
  - Blood culture
  - Urine culture
  - Spinal fluid culture in case of meningitis

Literature:

1. *Avendano J, Tanishima T, Kuwabara T:* Ocular cryptococcosis. Am J Ophthalmol 86: 110–113, 1978
2. *Condon PI, Terry SI, Falconer H:* Cryptococcal eye disease. Doc Ophthalmol 44: 49–56, 1977
3. *Shields JA, Wright DW, Augsburger JJ, Wolkowicz MJ:* Cryptococcal chorioretinitis. Am J Ophthalmol 89: 210–218, 1980

3.49 Tuberculosis

Etiology:

- Infection by Mycobacterium tuberculosis, rarely by M. bovis or M. avis
- Inhalation of the pathogens into the lung
- Lymphatic or hematogenous distribution
- Histopathologically: granulomatous inflammation

General involvement:

- Primary lung involvement in 90%, followed by:
  - Development of a quiescent tuberculosis which can become activated

- Lymphogenous or hematogenous spread into the lymph nodes, pleura, urogenital system, bones and joints, lungs (miliary tuberculosis), meningeal membranes, peritoneum, eyes
  - Complete recovery
- Course depends on the patient's own resistance, among other things

Ocular involvement:

- Granulomatous and non-granulomatous iridocyclitis:
  - Rarely with tuberculoma in the anterior chamber
  - Usually chronic or with frequent acute recurrences
- Unifocal or multifocal choroiditis:
  - Usually bilateral
  - The spots have a diameter of 0.2–0.5 PD
  - Few spots, but in miliary tuberculosis there are many
  - Convalescence leaves behind pigmented scars
  - Development of a subretinal neovascularization membrane is possible
  - Possible transition to endophthalmitis
- Choroidal tuberculoma:
  - Intraocular, well-vascularized granuloma
  - Especially in miliary tuberculosis
- Vasculitis:
  - Periphlebitis
  - Rarely, occlusion of the central retinal vein
- Necrotizing retinochoroiditis:
  - Gray, rapidly growing spot
  - Massive vitreous and anterior chamber reaction
- Endophthalmitis:
  - Metastatic, subacute
  - Can develop from an iridocyclitis or choroiditis
- Uvea involvement in 48%, retinal involvement in 13%
- Other ocular manifestations:
  - Conjunctivitis (4%), sometimes phlyctenular

- Keratitis (26%)
- Scleritis, anterior and posterior (9%)

Diagnosis:

- History: history of family illnesses, immunosuppression, steroids
- X-ray diagnosis:
  - Beware: Negative results do not exclude tuberculosis
- Laboratory tests: direct demonstration of pathogens:
  - In gastric fluid or sputum
  - In aqueous and anterior chamber puncture specimens
- Tuberculin test:
  - Tine test, 5 IU tuberculin GT, or:
  - Intradermal injection of 5, 100 or 250 IU tuberculin GT
  - A skin reaction in the area of induration at least 10 mm in diameter is considered positive
  - Negative reaction: tuberculosis negative (15–20% are false-negative!) or anergy (e.g. in sarcoidosis) or reduction of the reaction through simultaneous corticosteroid therapy
  - Positive reaction: tuberculosis or false-positive (after BCG inoculation)

Remarks:

An immunosuppressive disease should always be considered as the basis for tuberculosis (HIV test). Iris granulomas should invariably arouse suspicion of tuberculosis or sarcoidosis. If all tests are inconclusive, a biopsy should be considered.

Literature:

1. *Coles RS:* Uveitis associated with systemic diseases. Surv Ophthalmol 8: 377–392, 1963
2. *Gur S, Silverstone BZ, Zilberman R, et al:* Chorioretinitis and extrapulmonary tuberculosis. Ann Ophthalmol 19: 112–115, 1987
3. *Helm CJ, Holland GN:* Ocular tuberculosis. Surv Ophthalmol 38: 229–256, 1993

3.50 Leprosy

Etiology:

- Caused by Myobacterium leprae infection
- The state of activity of the immune system determines the clinical picture:
  - Tuberculoid type: formation of granulomas (T-cell-dependent reaction)
  - Lepromatous type: bacteremia in the suppressed immune system
  - Indeterminate type: transitional stage between tuberculoid and lepromatous form
  - Borderline type: tuberculoid and lepromatous changes coexist for some time

General involvement:

- Tuberculoid form:
  - Skin: paresthetic, hypopigmented, sharply delimited plaques
  - Nervous system: paresthesia of peripheral nerves with muscular atrophy and contractures
- Lepromatous form:
  - Skin: plaques less well delimited
  - Involvement of all organs through bacteremia
  - Erythema nodosum

Ocular involvement:

- Ocular involvement in 20–100% of cases, especially in the lepromatous form
- Keratitis (typical, but possibly sometimes induced by simultaneous trachoma)
- Loss of eyebrows and eyelashes
- Lagophthalmos through affection of the facial nerve
- Lepromas (granulomas) on the lids
- Episcleritis, scleritis

- Optic nerve atrophy
- Anterior uveitis
  - Painless granulomas ('leprosy pearls'), i.e. iridocyclitis due to M. leprae's preference for the cooler, anterior parts of the eye
  - Infiltration of the pars plana
- Rarely, panuveitis
- Vasculitis

Diagnosis:
- Direct demonstration of the pathogen:
  - e.g. by iris biopsy using special staining techniques
- Lepromin test:
  - Skin reaction 48 hours after injection of 0.1 ml lepromin (extract of lepromatous tissue) is indicative of the tuberculoid type
  - Formation of violet nodules after 4 weeks can occur

Remarks:
Although lepromatous uveitis is rare at European and American latitudes, it still represents a common cause of blindness. Today there are 10-15 million people suffering from leprosy.

Literature:

1. *Brandt F, Malla OK:* Ocular findings in leprous patients. Graefe's Arch klin Ophthalmol 217: 27-34, 1981
2. *Espiritu CG, Gelber R, Ostler HB:* Chronic anterior uveitis in leprosy: an insidious cause of blindness. Br J Ophthalmol 75: 273-275, 1991
3. *Spaide R, Nattis R, Lipka A, D'Amico R:* Ocular findings in leprosy in the United States. Am J Ophthalmol 100: 411-416, 1985

3.51 Lues (syphilis)

Etiology:

- Infection by Treponema pallidum
- Transepithelial intake leads to bacteremia after an incubation period of a few weeks
- Congenital syphilis through placental transmission or infection during birth
- Increasing incidence, especially in immunodeficient patients (e.g. AIDS)

General involvement:

- Acquired syphilis:
  - Primary stage:
    - Primary chancre at the portal of entry (genital, oral)
    - Painless swelling of lymph nodes 1 week after the skin lesion
  - Secondary stage
    - 3-6 weeks thereafter, generalized lymphadenopathy from hematogenous dissemination, with fever, malaise, arthritic pain, weight loss, meningism
    - Skin changes (90 %):
      - Oral region (35 %)
      - Genital region (20 %)
      - Localized hair loss
    - Occasionally hepatitis, nephropathy
  - Latent stage:
    - Years to decades
    - No clinical symptoms
    - Serologic tests usually continue to be positive, spinal fluid unremarkable
  - Tertiary stage:
    - In 20% of untreated syphilis
    - Diffuse mild inflammation, but also:
    - Degeneration and necrosis

- Cardiovascular: aortitis
  - CNS: neurosyphilis (asymptomatic in 30%), tabes dorsalis, gummas
- Congenital syphilis:
  - Manifestation within 2–10 weeks, occasionally earlier or later
  - Development of Hutchinson's triad: saddle nose, Hutchinson teeth, keratitis
  - Periostitis
  - CNS anomalies
  - In severe cases: lymphadenopathy, anemia, jaundice, hepatosplenomegaly

Ocular involvement:

- Primary stage:
  - Conjunctival and blepharal chancre
- Secondary stage:
  - Syphilids: white painless conjunctival or scleral nodules
  - Iridocyclitis:
    - Occasionally granulomatous, usually fulminant
  - Localized iris inflammation:
    - Roseola iritis: diffuse hyperemia of the iris; remission after a few days or transition to:
    - Iritis papulosa: nodules in the pupillary zone which remit after some weeks, leaving atrophic, depigmented areas
  - Chorioretinitis:
    - Develops in the secondary stage in 50 % of patients
    - Uncharacteristic, diffuse or disseminated form
    - Marked vitreal reaction
    - Swelling of the optic nerve, edema of the posterior pole
    - Venous stasis
    - Obliterative vasculitis, especially of the arteries
    - Perivascular cotton-wool spots
    - Retinal hemorrhages
    - Exudative retinal detachment

    - Convalescence leaves behind pseudopigmentosa-like scars or leads to fibrotic transformation
    - Usually bilateral
  - Retinitis:
    - Two patterns are known:
      - Yellowish-white foci of retinitis outside the vascular arcade (with severe irritation of the anterior chamber) or
      - Grayish-white ring-shaped or map-like retinitis (at the level of the pigment epithelium) of the posterior pole
      - Normally unilateral
      - Particularly rapid course in immunosuppressed patients (e.g. AIDS) (cf. Chapter 3.26)
  - Neuroretinitis:
    - Primary involvement of the optic disc and retina
      - Papillitis, later optic disc atrophy
      - Occasionally with meningitis
      - With or without choroiditis
    - Pupil: Argyll-Robertson pupil syndrome
    - Lens: dislocation on account of defective ciliary zonules
- Congenital syphilis
  - Interstitial keratitis with vascularization
  - Keratouveitis
  - Iridocyclitis
  - Chororetinitis (14%):
    - 'Salt and pepper fundus'
    - Old scars (pigment hypertrophy or white areas)
    - Vitreal reaction
    - Possible formation of subretinal neovascularization membranes

Diagnosis:

- History:
  - Not always helpful, as the eye may be the only affected organ
  - Consultative examinations are required

- Clinical picture:
  - Iris changes are very characteristic, but apparently rare
  - 'Salt and pepper fundus' not pathognomonic (also found after, e.g., herpes simplex, varicella, rubella or mumps infections)
- Laboratory tests:
  - Direct demonstration of the pathogen: irrelevant to the diagnosis of uveitis
  - VDRL (Venereal Disease Research Laboratory) test:
    - Reveals antilipoidal antibodies
    - Suitable only as a screening test
    - Titer drops upon treatment
    - Often false-negative in the primary and latent stages
    - False-positive: pregnancy, advanced age, mononucleosis, leprosy
  - Demonstration of antibodies:
    - FTA-ABS (Fluorescent Treponemal Antibody Absorption) test:
      - Demonstration of anti-Treponema-pallidum antibodies
      - The test is positive in the primary and all later stages
      - Possibly false-positive in rheumatoid arthritis, lupus erythematosus, genital herpes infection, sometimes also in borreliosis
  - If there is serologic evidence of syphilis: examination of the cerebrospinal fluid to exclude neurosyphilis
  - If the serum tests lues-positive, it should also be tested for HIV, as there is an increasing coincidence of lues and AIDS

Remarks:

- Exclusion of syphilis is always mandatory in uveitis and can be done satisfactorily in the initial stage using the VDRL and FTA-ABS tests.
- The extent of possible cross-reactions with Borrelia burgdorferi has yet to be established with certainty. The ophthalmolo-

gic spectrum of clinical symptoms in the two diseases is probably very similar.

- An endemic form of syphilis (Bejel) is known in hot desert regions and probably leads to the same ocular symptoms as the venereally transmitted form, but to markedly less systemic changes (possibly no neurosyphilis and no cardiovascular complications); it probably does not occur congenitally either.

Literature:

1. *Arruga J, Valentines J, Mauri F, et al:* Neuroretinitis in acquired syphilis. Ophthalmology 92:262-270, 1985
2. *Mendelsohn AD, Jampol LM:* Syphilitic retinitis. Retina 4: 221-224, 1984
3. *Schlaegel TF Jr, Kao SF:* A review (1970-1980) of 28 presumptive cases of syphilitic uveitis. Am J Ophthalmol 93: 412-414, 1982
4. *Tamesis RR, Foster CS:* Ocular syphilis. Ophthalmology 97: 1281-1287, 1990

3.52 Lyme disease

Etiology:

- Infection by Borrelia burgdorferi
- Transmission by tick bite

General involvement:

- Stage 1:
  - Erythema chronicum migrans
  - Lymphadenopathy, fever, influenza-like symptoms
- Stage 2:
  - Erythema chronicum migrans, lymphocytoma (purple nodules, e.g. on the external ear or thorax)
  - Cardiac dysrhythmia, myocarditis
  - Arthralgia, especially of the knees
  - Meningitis, neuritis of the cranial nerves, radiculopathy, encephalitis

- Stage 3:
  - Acrodermatitis chronica atrophicans
  - Arthritis
  - Demyelinating encephalomyelitis, apoplexy, dementia

Ocular involvement:

- Stage 1:
  - Conjunctivitis
- Stage 2:
  - Anterior uveitis
  - Pars planitis
  - Choroiditis
  - Panuveitis
  - Panophthalmitis
  - Optic nerve neuritis
  - Horner's syndrome
  - Argyll-Robertson pupil syndrome
- Stage 3:
  - Interstitial keratitis
  - Episcleritis
  - Myositis

Diagnosis:

- History:
  - Tick bite (only recalled by 10% of patients)
  - Erythema chronicum migrans (ECM)
  - Previous knee complaints
- Clinical picture: in absence of ECM the clinical picture can be very uncharacteristic
- Laboratory tests:
  - Demonstration of antibodies
    - Immunofluorescence or ELISA assay:
      - IgM: proof of recent infection; however, test results are still negative in the early stage and return to negative after a few months

    - IgG: remains positive; the course of the titer can be revealing
  - Western blot test
    - In case of doubt, e.g., when syphilis cannot be serologically excluded
  - Cross-reactions occur between syphilis and borreliosis and can cause diagnostic problems; the most important criterion for differentiation seems to be a clearly positive FTA-ABS in lues serology

Remarks:

- Stage 1 Lyme disease may not show up clinically.
- Serologic testing is still beset with problems, since different laboratories use different antigen preparations and different methods of absorbing cross-reacting antibodies, so that there are no generally accepted standards.
- Because seronegative cases of Lyme disease have been reported, it seems advisable to adopt the view of the majority of clinicians, who refrain from speaking of ocular disease caused by Lyme disease unless there are clinical signs of systemic involvement.

Literature:

1. *Bialasiewicz AA, Ruprecht KW, Naumann GOH, Blenk H:* Bilateral diffuse choroiditis and exudative retinal detachment with evidence of Lyme disease. Am J Ophthalmol 105: 419-420, 1988
2. *Steere AC, Duray PH, Kauffmann DJH, Wormser GP:* Unilateral blindness caused by infection with the Lyme spirochete, Borrelia burgdorferi. Ann Intern Med 103: 382-385, 1985
3. *Winterkorn JMS:* Lyme disease: neurologic and ophthalmic manifestations. Survey Ophthalmol 35: 191-204, 1990

3.53 Whipple's disease

Etiology:

- An infectious (bacterial?) origin seems likely
- Middle-aged men account for 80–90% of patients

General involvement:

- Diarrhea, malabsorption, abdominal complaints
- Weight loss, fever, coughing, lymphadenopathy
- Hyperpigmentation of the skin
- Arthralgia after months or years (60–70%)
- CNS involvement (10%)
- Favorable prognosis

Ocular involvement:

- Episcleritis, scleritis
- Muscular pareses (with CNS involvement)
- Iridocyclitis
- Diffuse vasculitis:
  - Hemorrhages, exudates
  - Retinal capillary occlusion
  - Choroidal folds

Diagnosis:

- Clinical picture
- Biopsy:
  - From jejunal mucosa or vitreous
  - Shows PAS-positive staining of bacteroid structures in macrophages

Literature:

1. *Avila MP, Jalkh AE, Feldman E, et al:* Manifestations of Whipple's disease in the posterior segment of the eye. Arch Ophthalmol 102: 384–390, 1984

2. *Font RL, Rao NA, Issarescu St, McEntee WJ:* Ocular involvement in Whipple's disease. Arch Ophthalmol 96: 1431-1436, 1978
3. *Selsky EJ, Knox DL, Maumenee AE, Green WR:* Ocular involvement in Whipple's disease. Retina 4: 103-106, 1984

3.54 Endogenous bacterial endophthalmitis

Etiology:

- Metastatic in case of bacterial sepsis
- Microemboli enter ocular structures via the ocular blood vessels
- Predisposing factors:
  - Immunosuppression (malignancy, steroid treatment)
  - Antibody deficiency
  - In neonates
  - Diabetes mellitus
  - Cardiac disease
  - Renal failure
  - Postoperative period
  - Drug addiction
- Spectrum of pathogens:
  - Streptococcus pneumoniae
  - Streptococcus sp.
  - Bacillus cereus (esp. in drug addicts)
  - Listeria monocytogenes
  - Clostridium perfringens
  - Neisseria meningitis
  - Staphylococcus aureus (esp. following skin infection and in chronic systemic disease such as diabetes mellitus, renal failure)
  - Hemophilus influenzae
  - Actinobacillus sp.
  - Escherichia coli (with urogenital infection, in diabetes mellitus)

- Klebsiella pneumoniae
- Serratia marcescens
- Salmonella sp.
- Pseudomonas aeruginosa
- Proteus sp.
- Nocardia asteroides (esp. in immunosuppressed patients with pulmonary involvement)
- Myobacterium tuberculosis

- Endogenous forms account for 6–15% of all endophthalmitis
- Bilateral in ca. 25% (esp. Meningococcus, Escherichia coli, Klebsiella)
- Fulminant course: Pseudomonas, Streptococcus, Clostridium, Serratia, Neisseria (usually with meningitis), Hemophilus (often with meningitis)
- Slow course: Propionibacter acnes
- Indolent course: Listeria

General involvement:

- Origin of the bacterial microemboli:
  - Meningitis
  - Endocarditis
  - Urogenital system
  - Gastrointestinal tract
  - Skin, superficial wounds
  - Lung
  - Joints
  - Upper respiratory tract

Ocular involvement:

- Classification by location (1):
  - Anterior focal endophthalmitis:
    - Iritis (microabscess)
    - Severe irritation of the anterior chamber, possibly with hypopyon
    - Possible moderate vitreous opacification

    - Possible mild eyelid edema
  - Posterior focal endophthalmitis (retinitis septica):
    - Focal choroidal or retinal spots
    - Vitreous is moderately, sometimes severely infiltrated
    - Possible mild eyelid edema with ptosis
  - Diffuse anterior endophthalmitis:
    - Massive anterior chamber reaction with hypopyon
    - Iris usually cannot be evaluated
    - Pronounced corneal opacification
    - Conjunctival injection, blepharedema
    - Secondary glaucoma
    - Moderate vitreal infiltration
  - Diffuse posterior endophthalmitis:
    - Originates in posterior focal endophthalmitis
    - Retinitis
    - Arteriovascular occlusions
    - Massive vitreal reaction
    - Moderate to marked reaction of the anterior chamber
    - Moderate to marked inflammatory conjunctival injection
    - Often blepharedema, ptosis
    - Occasional secondary glaucoma
  - Panophthalmitis:
    - Exophthalmos, motility impairment
    - Blepharedema, ptosis
    - Massive inflammatory conjunctival injection, corneal opacification
    - Massive irritation of the anterior chamber with hypopyon
    - Severe yellowish-white vitreal infiltration
    - Retinal necrosis
    - Secondary glaucoma
- Retinal periphlebitis appears to be an early sign of staphylococcal endophthalmitis
- Prognosis:
  - Depends on the bacterium involved as well as on initial vision at the time of diagnosis and the time of vitrectomy

- Unfavorable:
  - Especially in panophthalmitis
  - In Bacillus cereus endophthalmitis

Diagnosis:

- History: Search for predisposing factors
- Laboratory tests:
  - Direct identification of the pathogen:
    - Blood culture
    - Urine culture
    - Spinal fluid culture in meningitis
    - Anterior chamber puncture
    - Diagnostic vitrectomy
    - Optimal: puncture of the anterior chamber and vitreous (positive results in 54-77% of cases)
    - Conjunctival culture is probably worthless

Remarks:

Although the incidence of metastatic endophthalmitis has generally decreased, it has risen in individual high-risk groups (drug addicts).

Literature:

1. *Greenwald MJ, Wohl LG, Sell CH:* Metastatic bacterial endophthalmitis: a contemporary reappraisal. Surv Ophthalmol 31: 81-101, 1986
2. *Hemady R, Zaltas M, Paton B, Foster CS, Baker AS:* Bacillus-induced endophthalmitis: new series of 10 cases and review of the literature. Br J Ophthalmol 74: 26-29, 1990
3. *Puliafito CA:* Endophthalmitis: advances in diagnosis and therapy. Curr Op Infect Dis 3: 559-562, 1990
4. *Rowsey JJ, Newsom DL, Sexton DJ:* Clinical diagnosis of endophthalmitis. Intl Ophthalmol Clin 27: 82-88, 1987

F) Systemic diseases and other forms of vasculitis

3.55 Sarcoidosis

Etiology:

- Unknown
- Diverse microorganisms have been suggested as pathogens
- Unknown antigens activate macrophages, thus interfering with T-cell (and consequently B-cell) regulation

General involvement:

- Presentation at first examination:
  - 20% asymptomatic
  - 50% with respiratory changes
  - 25% with symptoms such as fever, nausea, weight loss
  - 5% with extrathoracic symptoms
- Overall involvement:
  - Joint and muscular involvement: polyarticular arthritis, bone lesions, myositis, progressive myopathy, typical children's form (under 5 years) of polyarthritis
  - Peripheral lymphadenopathy
  - Skin symptoms: erythema nodosum, lupus pernio, subcutaneous skin nodules, thickening and purple coloring of scars
  - Neurologic symptoms (5% of patients): cranial neuropathy (esp. of the 7th cranial nerve), opticoneuropathy (ca. 12%), aseptic meningitis, peripheral neuropathy
  - Cardiac symptoms: arrhythmia, pericarditis
  - Renal symptoms: kidney stones, nephrosclerosis due to hypercalcemia
  - Other organs: hepatomegaly (20%), rise in alkaline phosphatase (30-40%), splenomegaly (up to 40%), bone marrow infiltration with granulomas (15-40%)

Ocular involvement:

- In 25-30% of patients with histologically confirmed sarcoidosis

- In 2% the eye is the only organ involved
- Lacrimal gland involvement in 50% of patients (gallium scan)
- Anterior uveitis (22–70%):
  - Iris granulomas are possible
- Posterior uveitis (14–43%):
  - 'Candle wax' phenomena on retinal vessels in some cases
  - More often, white dots of various sizes (multifocal choroiditis)
  - Rarely, large choroidal granulomas
- Pars planitis (ca. 10%)
- Vasculitis (10–17%):
  - Mostly venous vessels involved

Diagnosis:

- History and clinical picture
- Chest X-ray
- Gallium scanning (probably the most sensitive test)
- Bronchoalveolar lavage
- Laboratory tests: determination of serum ACE
- Confirmation by histologic ocular examination, e.g. via conjunctival biopsy or, less frequently, lacrimal gland biopsy
- The Kveim provocation test is not practical and may transmit infectious diseases

Remarks:

- Sarcoidosis is one of the chameleons in the diagnosis of uveitis
- Gallium scanning currently appears to be the most sensitive method. However, because of the radiation exposure involved, it should be reserved for patients in whom histologic or radiologic confirmation of the disease is pending despite suspected sarcoidosis uveitis (e.g. in granulomatous uveitis, possibly pars planitis, typical chorioretinitis, borderline or elevated ACE levels).
- Absence of pulmonary involvement under X-ray examination appears not to exclude sarcoidosis uveitis. Even if tests for sar-

coidosis give negative results, they should be repeated at intervals of 1-2 years in recurrent uveitis.

- It appears important to identify sarcoidosis as a possible cause of uveitis, since it has been the experience of many uveitis specialists that corticosteroids are the best therapy for sarcoidosis-uveitis.

Literature:

1. *Jabs DA, Johns CJ:* Ocular involvement in chronic sarcoidosis. Am J Ophthalmol 102: 297-301, 1986
2. *Karma A, Huhti E, Poukkula A:* Course and outcome of ocular sarcoidosis. Am J Ophthalmol 106: 467-472, 1988
3. *Mayers M:* Ocular sarcoidosis. Int Ophthalmol Clin 30: 257-263, 1990
4. *Zierhut M, Foster CS:* Multiple sclerosis, sarcoidosis and other diseases in patients with pars planitis. Böke WRF, Manthey KF, Nussenblatt RB (Editors): Intermediate Uveitis. Dev Ophthalmol, Vol. 23, Basel, Karger, 1992, pp. 41-47

3.56 Behçet's disease

Etiology:

- Unknown
- Environmental influences of a viral (e.g. HSV), bacterial (e.g. streptococci) or toxic origin have been suggested as possible causes
- A genetic component seems to be involved, because in Japan, Mediterranean countries and some countries in Europe the association with HLA-B51 is high (50-70% vs. 12% in healthy subjects); interestingly, this has not been confirmed for America.
- The highest incidence is found in countries along the Silk Road (from the Mediterranean Sea via Turkey to Japan)
- Histopathologically, obliterative vasculitis is typical

General involvement:

- Oral ulcers (99%)
- Ulcers in the genital region (78%)
- Further skin lesions (75%): erythema nodosum, vesiculopapular eruptions
- Arthritis (especially of the knee and ankle joints) (60%)
- Thrombophlebitis (10–20%) (in Europe, 73% has been reported)
- Gastrointestinal complaints (abdominal pain, diarrhea, constipation)
- Ulcerative enterocolitis
- Involvement of the central nervous system: meningitis, pareses, epileptiform attacks and many other symptoms
- Epididymitis
- Rarely, renal involvement

Ocular involvement:

- Conjunctivitis, subconjunctival hemorrhages
- Episcleritis, scleritis
- Keratitis
- Iridocyclitis
  - With or without hypopyon
  - Often bilateral
- Choroiditis
- Retinal hemorrhages, edema, exudates, serous retinal detachment, possibly with accompanying vitritis
- Swelling of the optic nerve, hyperemia, atrophy
- Vasculitis of small veins and arteries: sheathing, arterial vasoconstriction with venous stasis, branch or central vein occlusion
- Myositis
- Ocular involvement in 70–85% of cases

Diagnosis:

- Diagnostic criteria (Japanese criteria):

- Recurrent oral ulcers (at least 3 times in one year)
- In addition at least 2 of the following 4 criteria:
  - Recurrent genital ulcers
  - Ocular involvement: uveitis or retinal vasculitis
  - Skin lesions: erythema nodosum, pseudofolliculitis or papulopustular changes or
  - Acneform nodules not attributable to steroids
- Other diagnostic criteria seem to be equivalent (1)

- Clinical picture and history
- Pathergy test:
  - Prick test or
  - Intradermal injection of saline solution
  - Leads to distinct redness and swelling of the tested area within 48 hours
- Fluorescein angiography:
  - Early phase: small focal fluorescein leaks in the macula; these are an important diagnostic criterion
- Electrophysiology:
  - ERG may already exhibit changes at an early stage

Remarks:

The clinical picture of Behçet's disease in Japan appears to be much more severe and different in some respects to the one found in Europe and America. Whereas anterior forms of uveitis are also found in Behçet's disease in Japan, vasculitic involvement of the posterior segments and thromboembolic events in other parts of the body are the rule in Europe and the United States.

Literature:

1. *International study group for Behçet's disease:* Criteria for diagnosis of Behçet's disease. Lancet 335: 1078-1080, 1990
2. *Michelson JB, Friedlaender MH:* Behçet's disease. Int Ophthalmol Clin 30: 271-278, 1990
3. *Kötter I, Dürk H, Fierlbeck G,et al.:* Behcet's disease in 39 German and Mediterranean patients. In: Godeau P, Wechs-

ler B (editors). Behcet's Disease. Elsevier Science Publishers, Amsterdam, 1993, pp. 197-200

3.57 Uveitis in multiple sclerosis

Etiology:

- Pathogenesis unclear
- Autoimmune etiology induced by a virus is possible
- Genetic factors appear important (HLA-DR2 or HLA-DRw6, both in combination with HLA-DQw1b), but this cannot yet be determined routinely

General involvement:

- Demyelination and accompanying inflammation lead to paralytic symptoms, depending on the affected area
- Recurrent, usually chronic progressive course
- Remission or arrest of the disease can occur

Ocular involvement:

- Optic nerve neuritis (40%)
- Cranial nerve pareses, internuclear ophthalmoplegia, nystagmus
- Anterior uveitis
- Pars planitis:
  - 8-11% of patients with pars planitis have MS
  - 3-27% of MS patients develop pars planitis
  - Clinical signs can precede MS by many years
  - Occasionally associated with optic nerve neuritis and/or retinal periphlebitis
- Retinal periphlebitis (6-8%):
  - Mild, often asymptomatic
- Retinitis (ca. 20%):
  - Independent of retinal vessels
  - Intraretinal foci 1-2 mm in size
  - Usually asymptomatic
- Panuveitis (2-5%)

Diagnosis:

- Definition (2, 3):
  - Clinically confirmed:
    - More than one lesion confirmed or
    - Two anamnestic episodes, one lesion and changes in visually evoked potentials (VEP) or lesions confirmed by NMR
  - Confirmed diagnosis, supported by laboratory tests:
    - Two lesions, either anamnestic or upon examination or
    - One lesion, either anamnestic or upon examination, and, in addition, one episode, a lesion confirmed by changed VEP or NMR, and an abnormal gammaglobulin concentration in the spinal fluid
  - Clinically suspect:
    - Two lesions, either anamnestic or suggested upon examination

Remarks:

HLA results obtained by molecular biologic methods appear very promising; however, they have been obtained from MS patients in whom possible ocular symptoms were not taken into account.

Literature:

1. *Arnold AC, Pepose JS, Hepler RS Foos RY:* Retinal periphlebitis and retinitis in multiple sclerosis. Ophthalmology 91: 255-262, 1984
2. *Poser CM:* The course of multiple sclerosis. Arch Neurol 42: 1035, 1985
3. *Schumacher GA, Beebe G, Kibler RF et al.:* Problems of experimental trials of therapy in multiple sclerosis. Ann NY Acad Sci 122: 552-568, 1965
4. *Wagemans MAJ, Breebart AC:* Association between intermediate uveitis and multiple sclerosis. In: Böke WRF, Manthey KF, Nussenblatt RB (Editors): Intermediate Uveitis. Dev Ophthalmol. Karger, Basel, Vol. 23, pp. 99-105, 1992

5. *Zierhut M, Foster CS:* Multiple sclerosis, sarcoidosis and other diseases in patients with pars planitis. In: Böke WRF, Manthey KF, Nussenblatt RB (Editors): Intermediate Uveitis. Dev Ophthalmol Karger, Basel, Vol. 23, pp. 41–47, 1992

3.58 Systemic lupus erythematosus

Etiology:

- Unknown
- Dysfunction of the T-cell system leads, among other things, to dysregulation of the B-lymphocytes followed by autoantibody production
- Immune complexes of these autoantigen-autoantibodies lead to typical vasculitis of small vessels
- The resulting activation of proteolytic enzymes and neutrophilic granulocytes, among other cells, leads to tissue damage
- Occasionally induced by drugs
- Genetic predisposition is possible
- Classification according to the extent of involvement into:
  - Discoid form
  - Systemic lupus erythematosus (SLE)
  - Special forms of SLE:
    - Primary antiphospolipid syndrome
    - Sneddon's disease

General involvement:

- Discoid lupus (limited to the skin in 90% of patients)
- SLE:
  - Arthralgia or arthritis (92%)
  - Skin involvement (72%), acute (= butterfly rash)
  - Renal involvement (53%)
  - Myalgia (48%)
  - Pleuritis (45%)
  - CNS involvement (26%)
  - General symptoms (fever, anorexia, vomiting, nausea) (50-85%)

- Primary antiphospholipid syndrome
  - CNS involvement (stroke, atypical migraine, chorea, transient ischemic attacks)
  - Thromboses (thrombosis of the deep leg veins, mesenteric renal or cardiac vessels, pulmonary embolism, peripheral arteries)
  - Livedo racemosa (Sneddon's disease)
  - Typically seen in young people

Ocular involvement:

- Discoid form:
  - Erythema, telangiectasia of the eyelids
  - Blepharoconjunctivitis (good site for biopsy!)
  - Conjunctivitis, possibly ulcerative
  - Rarely keratitis
  - Sicca syndrome
- SLE:
  - Erythema of the eyelids
  - Conjunctivitis
  - Keratoconjunctivitis sicca, stromal keratitis
  - Episcleritis, scleritis
  - Accommodation problems, homonymous hemianopsia, internuclear ophthalmoplegia, nystagmus, ptosis
  - Papilledema, optic neuritis, optic ischemia, atrophy
  - Anterior uveitis, usually presenting as sclerouveitis
  - Retinal vasculitis:
    - Focal ischemia with cotton-wool spots
    - Intraretinal hemorrhages
    - Absence of papilledema
    - This form takes a mild course
    - May be indistinguishable from fundus hypertonicus
    - Occlusive vasculitis, usually of the arterioles or venules
    - Proliferative retinopathy on rare occasions with ischemia-induced neovascularization, intraretinal hemorrhages, possibly also vitreal bleeding, frequently with
    - Optic nerve involvement

- Antiphospholipid syndrome
  - Transient diplopia, homonymous visual field defect
  - Unilateral or bilateral obliterative retinopathy
  - Retinal neovascularization, vitreal bleeding
  - Ischemic optic neuropathy
  - In severe retinal changes: CNS involvement in 73% of cases

Diagnosis:

- Classification of SLE (4) is based on 11 criteria, of which at least four should be present over the entire observation period:
  - Butterfly rash: facial except for the nasolabial area (in 30% of patients)
  - Discoid erythema
  - Photosensitivity: erythema after normal exposure to sunlight
  - Oral or nasopharyngeal ulcers
  - Non-destructive arthritis affecting at least two sites
  - Pleuritis or pericarditis
  - Renal involvement: persistent proteinuria (>0.5 g/d) or urinary casts or pathologic urinary cytology
  - Neurologic involvement: convulsive disorders or psychoses
  - Hematologic involvement: hemolytic anemia or leukopenia or lymphopenia or thrombocytopenia
  - Immunologic findings: positive LE-cells or anti-DNA-antibody or anti-Sm-nuclear antibody or false-positive lues test after having been confirmed as positive for at least 6 months (FTA-ABS test or immobilization test)
  - Antinuclear antibodies
- Laboratory tests:
  - Antinuclear antibodies:
    - Positive in 99% of patients
    - Occasionally false-positive (cf. Chapter 1.3.4)
    - A homogeneous and diffuse staining pattern is typical
  - Anti-DNA-antibodies:

    - Typically anti-dsDNA (double-stranded) antibodies, which are practically pathognomonic for SLE
- Anti-Sm-antibodies:
    - Almost exclusively in SLE
- Anti-Ro(SS-A)-antibodies:
    - Found in various forms of lupus and in Sjögren's disease
- Antiphospholipid antibodies:
    - Found in Sneddon's disease and primary antiphospolipid syndrome, also in Huntington's chorea, Guillain-Barré syndrome and SLE (then high risk of cerebral infarct), Behçet's disease, AIDS, Lyme disease
    - Patients often test ANA-negative
- CH50:
    - Decrease of this total complement parameter reflects SLE activity
    - As this measurement is not solely typical of SLE it is only helpful if SLE-associated antibodies are also found
- Complement components C1, C4 and C2:
    - Congenital deficiencies of these components can trigger SLE

Remarks:
Scleritis and retinal vasculopathy are indicative of an active stage of the systemic disease. Amelioration of these symptoms is a good parameter for the success of the treatment.

Literature:

1. *Graham EM, Spalton DJ, Barnard RO, et al*: Cerebral and retinal vascular changes in systemic lupus erythematosus. Ophthalmology 92: 444-448, 1985
2. *Jonas J, Kölble K, Völcker HE, Kalden JR*: Central retinal artery occlusion in Sneddon disease associated with antiphospholipid antibodies. Am J Ophthalmol 102: 37-40, 1986
3. *Snyers B, Lambert M, Hardy JP*: Retinal and choroidal vaso-occlusive disease in systemic lupus erythematosus associated with antiphospholipid antibodies. Retina 10: 255-260, 1990

4. *Tan EM, Cohen AS, Fries JF, et al*: The 1982 revised criteria for the classification of systemic lupus erythematosus. Arthritis Rheum 28: 1271-1277, 1982

3.59 Wegener's granulomatosis

Etiology:

- Unknown, an infectious etiology is currently presumed
- Leads to the release of lysosomal enzymes and activation of B- and T-lymphocytes
- Production of antibodies (ANCA among others) and development of vasculitis due to polyclonal B-cell activation
- Two forms:
  - Generalized: involvement of various organs with an unfavorable prognosis
  - Limited: involvement of usually only one organ system, frequently with a much more favorable prognosis

General involvement:

- Ear, nose and throat (95%):
  - Sinusitis, rhinitis, otitis media, ulceration, parotid swelling, nasal obstruction, septal perforation
- Lung (52%):
  - Tracheal stenosis, lung infiltration, cavern formation leading to cough, hemoptysis, bronchospasm
- Epicarditis, coronary arteritis, myocarditis
- Glomerulonephritis (80%), can progress rapidly but rarely leads to hypertension
- Arthritis (32%)
- Nervous system involvement (18%):
  - Cranial nerve pareses, CNS granulomas, peripheral neuropathies, paresthesia, signs of cerebral vasculitis
- Skin:
  - Petechial hemorrhages, purpura, ulceration, nodules

Ocular involvement:
- Pseudotumor of the orbit, erythematous blepharedema (50%)
- Ptosis
- Nasolacrimal obstruction, dacryocystitis (25%)
- Conjunctivitis
- Marginal keratitis (25%)
- Scleritis, episcleritis (25%), often with
- Anterior uveitis
- Pars planitis
- Panuveitis
- Occlusive retinal vasculitis
- Retinopathy (rare in the limited form):
  - Similar to that seen in arterial hypertension (but also found without hypertension)
  - Cotton-wool spots, hemorrhages
- Papilledema or secondary optic nerve involvement because of orbital involvement (20%)
- Ocular involvement in 40% of patients

Diagnosis:
- Clinical picture
- Laboratory tests:
  - cANCA (classical anti-neutrophilic cytoplasmic antibodies)
    - Nearly pathognomonic for Wegener's granulomatosis, but also found in 10-15% of uveitis patients without further signs of Wegener
    - Titer level correlates with the activity of the disease and thus serves as a measure of therapeutic efficacy
  - The relevance of pANCA (perinuclear ANCA) is unclear at the moment

Remarks:
- The easy availability of ANCA determination has increased the number of cases diagnosed and treated at an early stage.
- This and consistent immunosuppressive therapy has resulted

in a considerably improved prognosis of this otherwise lethal disease.

- Determination of cANCA should always be performed when there are signs of scleritis.

Literature:

1. *Bullen CL, Liesegang TJ, McDonald GJ, DeRemee RA*: Ocular complications of Wegener's granulomatosis. Ophthalmology 90: 279-290, 1983
2. *Duncker G, Beigel A, Lehmenn H*: Wegener'sche Granulomatose: okuläre Manifestationen, Diagnose und Therapie. Klin Mbl Augenheilk 181: 184-187, 1982
3. *Spalton DJ, Graham EM, Page NGR, Sanders MD*: Ocular changes in limited forms of Wegener's granulomatosis. Br J Ophthalmol 65: 553-563, 1981
4. *Wolff-Kormann PG, Stefani FH, Riedel KG*: Okuläre Frühsymptome bei Wegener-Granulomatose. Fortschr Ophthalmol 87: 488-491, 1990

3.60 Relapsing polychondritis

Etiology:

- Autoimmune disease, possibly a reaction to type II collagen
- The inducing agent is not known
- Histopathologically: granulomatous vasculitis
- Frequently in the context of other autoimmune diseases

General involvement:

- Inflammation of the auricle (85%)
- Involvement of the inner ear (39%)
- Inflammation of the nasal cartilage (63%)
- Arthropathies (70%)
- Laryngotracheobronchial involvement (51%)
- Skin involvement (26%)

Ocular involvement:

- Lid edema
- Keratitis (including sicca, defects)
- Episcleritis, scleritis (36%)
- Anterior uveitis (20%)
- Vasculitis of the retinal vessels
- Muscular pareses
- Optic nerve neuritis, papilledema
- Orbital infiltration
- Isaak et al. (4) report on 112 patients, 50% of whom had ocular symptoms and in 19% of whom these were the initial ocular manifestation

Diagnosis:

- Diagnostic criteria (according to (5), modified by (1)):
  - Three or more of the following symptoms:
    - Recurrent chondritis of both auricles
    - Chondritis of the nasal cartilage
    - Non-destructive polyarthritis
    - Inflammation of ocular structures
    - Chondritis of the respiratory tract
    - Cochlear or vestibular lesions, or:
  - One of the six criteria in addition to positive biopsy (vasculitis), or
  - Chondritis affecting at least two anatomical sites and responding to steroids or dapsone
- Clinical picture and history
- Laboratory tests:
  - Autoantibodies against cartilage (40%)
  - Anti-collagen-type-II antibodies (33%)
  - Antinuclear antibodies (25%)

Remarks:

Recurrent polychondritis is potentially lethal on account of its tracheal involvement, and has the same destructive effect on the eye as vasculitis of other etiology. There appears to be an overlap with Behçet's disease and possibly also with Wegener's granulomatosis (MAGIC syndrome) (2).

Literature:

1. *Damiani JM, Levine HL*: Relapsing polychondritis-report of ten cases. Laryngoscope 89: 929–944, 1979
2. *Firestein GS, Gruber HE, Weisman MH, Zvaifler NJ, Barber J, O'Duffy JD*: Mouth and genital ulcers with inflamed cartilage: MAGIC-Syndrome: JAMA 79: 65–72, 1985
3. *Hoang-Xuan T, Foster CS, Rice BA*: Scleritis in relapsing polychondritis. Ophthalmology 97: 892–898, 1990
4. *Isaak BL, Liesegang TJ, Michet CJ*: Ocular and systemic findings in relapsing polychondritis. Ophthalmology 93: 681–689, 1986
5. *McAdams LP, O'Hanlan MA, Bluestone R, Pearson DM*: Relapsing polychondritis: prospective study of 23 patients and a review of the literature. Medicine 55: 193–215, 1976
6. *Zierhut M, Foster CS:* Uveitis and relapsing polychondritis. In: Dernouchamps JP, Verougstraete C, Caspers-Velu L, Tassignon MJ (editors) Recent advances in uveitis. Kugler, Amsterdam, 1993, pp. 487–489

3.61 Polyarteritis nodosa

Etiology:

- Unknown
- Immune complex formation leads to vasculitis with ensuing necrosis of small and medium-sized arteries
- The hepatitis-B-surface antigen appears to be causally involved in the vasculitis
- Develops after hepatitis B-virus infection in one out of 500 cases
- Men are affected 3 times as often as women
- Occurs at all ages, but especially in people between 20 and 40 years of age

General involvement:

- Onset frequently with an infection, feeling of weakness, anorexia, fever, weight loss, joint complaints (75%)
- Leukocytosis, eosinophilia, anemia, ESR elevation (80%)
- Coronary arteritis or pericarditis (80%)
- Peripheral neuropathy (50-70%), often the initial symptom
- Renal involvement (65-80%), renal hypertension (25%)
- Abdominal pains, nausea, diarrhea, hemorrhages (60-75%)
- Purpura, skin ulcerations, livedo reticularis, fingertip infarctions
- Polyarthritis (20%)
- Epididymitis

Ocular involvement:

- Orbital pseudotumor
- Muscular pareses
- Episcleritis, scleritis
- Corneal ulceration
- Anterior uveitis
- Retinal vasculitis
- Ocular involvement in 20% of patients

Diagnosis:

- History and clinical picture: the eyes can be the site of the initial manifestation of the disease
- Laboratory tests: demonstration of hepatitis-B-surface antigen (positive in 30-40%)
- Biopsy: demonstration of vasculitis confirms the disease

Remarks:

A rare disease (incidence ca. 1 : 100,000)

Literature:

1. *Morgan CM, Foster CS, D'Amico DJ, Gragoudas ES*: Retinal vasculitis in polyarthritis nodosa. Retina: 6: 205-209, 1986

2. *Robin JB, Schanzlin DJ, Meisler DM, deLuise VP, Clough JD*: Ocular involvement in the respiratory vasculitides. Surv Ophthalmol 30: 127-140, 1985
3. *Solomon SM, Solomon JH*: Bilateral central artery occlusion in polyarteritis nodosa. Ann Ophthalmol 10: 567-569, 1978

3.62 Systemic sclerosis (scleroderma)

Etiology:

- Pathogenesis appears to involve collagen overproduction by fibroblasts, leading to the typical microvasculopathy
- Cytokines from activated mononuclear cells are thought to trigger the increased production of collagen
- Obliterated vessels due to microvasculopathy, with consequent dysfunction of the end organs
- There is no unequivocal genetic component
- 75-85% of patients are women
- Differentiation according to the extent of the sclerosis:
  - Systemic sclerosis (scleroderma):
    - With diffuse skin involvement (progressive systemic sclerosis, PSS)
    - With limited skin involvement (CREST syndrome)
  - Multiple forms (chemically induced, pseudosclerodermic forms, overlap syndromes) (for a review, see (4))

General involvement:

- PSS:
  - Esophageal motility disorders (75%)
  - Lung dysfunction (56%), interstitial fibrosis (44%)
  - Myopathy (20%)
  - Raynaud's syndrome (85%)
  - Arthralgias (80%)
  - Calcinosis cutis (5%)
  - Renal involvement (15%)
- CREST syndrome (most important differences compared with PSS):

- Calcinosis cutis (45%)
- Raynaud's syndrome (95%)
- Esophageal motility disorders (75%)
- Skin involvement (95%)
- Telangiectasias (80%)
- Involvement of the joints, kidneys and heart are somewhat rarer than in PSS

Ocular involvement:

- PSS:
  - Sicca syndrome (70%)
  - Progressive shortening of the conjunctival fornix (60%)
  - Episcleritis (5%)
  - Retinopathy and vascular changes of the choroid (50%):
    - Multiple non-perfused choroidal areas (50%)
    - Cotton-wool spots and intraretinal hemorrhages (as in arterial hypertension, which is also often found, though not always)
- CREST syndrome:
  - Sicca syndrome
  - Retinopathy is not known
- In the other forms ocular involvement is unclear

Diagnosis:

- Criteria for the diagnosis of scleroderma (2) (the main criterion or two of the subordinate criteria are required):
  - Main criterion:
    - Thickening, induration and hardening of the skin of the fingers and proximal to the metacarpal or metatarsal joints, sometimes all over the body
  - Subordinate criteria:
    - Sclerodactylia: changes limited to the fingers
    - Digital pitting scars or loss of substance at the tips of the fingers
      - Bibasilar pulmonary fibrosis, but not in the context of primary lung disease

- Laboratory tests:
  - Antibody determination:
    - Antinuclear antibodies: 55% in PSS, 50% in CREST
    - Anti-centromere antibodies: 5% in PSS, 50% in CREST
    - Scl-70 antibodies: 40% in PSS, 15% in CREST

Literature:

1. *Farkas TG, Sylvester V, Archer D*: The choroidopathy of progressive systemic sclerosis. Am J Ophthalmol 74: 875-886, 1972
2. *Masi AT, Rodnan GP, Medsger TA Jr, et al.*: Preliminary criteria for the classification of systemic sclerosis (scleroderma). Arthritis Rheum 23: 581-590, 1980
3. *Schumacher H Jr*: Systemic sclerosis and localized scleroderma. In: Schumacher H Jr (Editor). Primer on the rheumatic diseases, 9th ed., Arthritis Foundation, Atlanta, 1988, pp. 111-117

3.63 Dermatomyositis

Etiology:

- Unknown
- There is evidence of a viral etiology
- In rare cases drugs induce the disease
- There is a genetic component, since HLA-B8 and HLA-DR3 are more frequently found
- Immunopathogenesis via autoimmune disease is presumed, since numerous autoantibodies are detectable
- None of these antibodies appears responsible for the tissue lesions
- Vascular lesions following vasculitis lead to inflammation of the skin and muscles
- Designated as type II of idiopathic inflammatory muscular disease (polymyositis)
- Dermatomyositis during childhood is designated as type IV polymyositis

General involvement:

- Symmetric proximal muscular weakness
- Feeling of weakness, weight loss
- Skin involvement:
  - Exanthema (40%) on elbows, knees, ankles, backs of the fingers, and on the face
  - Hyperpigmented skin areas adjacent to hypopigmented areas
- Raynaud's syndrome
- Lung fibrosis (5-10%)
- Pericarditis, congestive heart failure, cardiac dysrhythmia (50%)
- Difficulty in swallowing, dysphagia, reflux
- Malignant tumors seem to occur 4-5 times more frequently than in normal individuals

Ocular involvement:

- Periorbital edema, ptosis
- Mauve discoloration of the eyelids (pathognomonic)
- Conjunctivitis
- Episcleritis, scleritis
- Peripheral corneal ulcers
- Muscular pareses
- Anterior uveitis
- Retinopathy as in hypertension (and sometimes caused by it)
- Retinal vasculitis
- Ischemic infarction of the choriocapillaris (Elschnig's bodies)
- Ischemic optic neuropathy
- Ocular changes in type II and type IV polymyositis

Diagnosis:

- Clinical picture
- Laboratory tests:
  - Elevated transaminase, creatinine kinase, lactate dehydrogenase and aldolase levels

- Electromyography for the exclusion of other muscular disease
- Muscular biopsy is decisive

Remarks:
Rare; incidence 1:1,000,000

Literature:

1. *Bruce GM:* Retinitis in dermatomyositis. Trans Am Ophthalmol Soc 36: 282–297, 1938
2. *Foster CS, Yee M:* Corneoscleral manifestations of Graves' disease, the acquired connective tissue disorders, and systemic vasculitis. Int Ophthalmol Clin 23: 131–157, 1983
3. *Otradovec J, Stieber V, Suta M:* Retinopathie bei Polymyositis. Klin Mbl Augenheilk 156: 498–507, 1970

3.64 Mucocutaneous Lymph Node Syndrome (Kawasaki's Disease)

Etiology:
- Unknown, possibly microbial (e.g. rickettsiae, Propionibacterium acnes, retroviruses)
- Systemic necrotizing arteritis of small and medium-sized vessels
- Children between 3 months and 12 years contract the disease (peak incidence in the 3rd–4th year of life)
- Occasionally epidemic, especially among Japanese children

General involvement:
- At the beginning, high fever without a prodromal stage
- Conjunctival congestion (90%) and redness of the lips, mucous membrane formation in the mouth, polymorphous exanthema on the trunk or extremities, redness of the palms and soles, occasionally cervical lymphadenopathy
- Mild pancarditis, coronary aneurysms (40%) receding to 3–5% after one year; coronary infarction can occur after thrombosis

- Symptoms disappear as fever goes down
- After 10–15 days, scaling of the skin of the fingers
- Other possible symptoms: diarrhea, abdominal pain, gallbladder hydrops, paralytic ileus, arthritis, aseptic meningitis, facial paralysis, hemiplegia, encephalopathy

Ocular involvement:
- Conjunctivitis
- Superficial keratitis
- Anterior uveitis (nearly always):
  - Acute, mild course
  - Usually during the first week of disease
- Papilledema
- Vasculitis (rare)

Diagnosis:
- Diagnostic criteria

  a) Five should be fulfilled:
  - Persistent fever lasting five days or longer
  - Peripheral extremities:
    - Initially: redness or edema of the palms and soles
    - During convalescence: membranous scaling of the fingertips
  - Polymorphous exanthema
  - Bilateral conjunctivitis
  - Redness of the lips, strawberry-colored tongue, diffuse redness of the oral and pharyngeal mucosa
  - Acute non-purulent cervical lymphadenopathy

  b) Or four of the above-listed criteria in addition to proven coronary aneurysm
- Laboratory tests: non-specific inflammatory signs

Remarks:
The disease appears to be very rare in Europe.

Literature:

1. *Krüger H, Poetzsch-Heffter R:* Ophthalmologische Nachuntersuchungen beim Kawasaki-Syndrom. Fortschr Ophthalmol 83: 181-183, 1986
2. *Mills MD, Smith LBH:* Kawasaki Syndrome. Int Ophthalmol Clin 32: 81-92, 1992
3. *Ohno S, Miyajima T, Higushi M, et al.:* Ocular manifestations of Kawasaki's disease (mucocutaneous lymph node syndrome). Am J Ophthalmol 93: 713-717, 1982

3.65 Allergic granulomatosis (Churg-Strauss syndrome)

Etiology:

- Unknown, possibly viral etiology
- Histopathologically, granulomatous necrotizing vasculitis of small vessels, often with eosinophilic infiltration
- Men are affected more often than women
- History usually includes asthma, allergic rhinitis or peripheral eosinophilia

General involvement:

- Pulmonary infiltrates (Loeffler's syndrome) before or at the onset of vasculitis
- Skin nodules, purpura, arthralgia, non-deforming arthritis
- Neuritis
- Hypertension
- Focal segmental glomerulonephritis
- Congestive heart failure
- 5-year-survival rate: 60%

Ocular involvement:

- Conjunctival granuloma
- Marginal corneal ulcers
- Episcleritis

- Retinal vasculitis
- Ischemic optic neuropathy

Diagnosis:

- Laboratory tests:
  - Leukocytosis with eosinophilia
  - Elevated ESR
  - Elevated serum IgE

Literature:

1. *Cury D, Breakey AS, Payne BF:* Allergic granulomatous angiitis associated with uveascleritis and papilledema. Arch Ophthalmol 55: 261-266, 1956
2. *Rabinowitz L, Currie J:* Branch retinal artery occlusion in the Churg-Strauss syndrome. J Clin Neuro Ophthalmol 5: 229-237, 1985
3. *Weinstein JM, Chui H, Lane S, et al.:* Churg-Strauss syndrome (allergic granulomatous angiitis). Arch Ophthalmol 101: 1217-1220, 1983

3.66 Takayasu's arteritis (pulseless disease)

Etiology:

- Unknown
- Histopathologically, granulomatous inflammation of the media and intima with occlusion of large arteries
- A genetic component seems possible (associated with HLA-Bw52 in Japan)
- Particularly high incidence among young Asian women
- Average age 30 years

General involvement:

- The disease begins with fever, anorexia, weight loss, myalgia, arthralgia and non-destructive arthritis (20%)
- Erythema-nodosum-like changes in the skin

- Arterial hypertension (40%), absence of pulsation, blue patches due to vascular occlusions
- Aortic aneurysms
- 5-year survival rate: 80%

Ocular involvement:
- Diplopia
- Episcleritis
- Anterior uveitis
- Hypertensive retinopathy, occasionally associated with neovascularization

Diagnosis:
- Laboratory tests
  - Erythrocyte sedimentation rate elevated during inflammatory stage
- Angiography reveals vascular occlusions

Remarks:
A rare disease.

Literature:

1. *Ishikawa K:* Natural history and classification of occlusive thromboaortopathy (Takayasu's disease). Circulation 57: 27-35, 1978
2. *Shelhammer JH, Volkman DJ, Parillo JE, et al.:* Takayasu's arteritis and its therapy. Ann Intern Med 103: 121-126, 1985

3.67 Thrombangiitis obliterans (Buerger's disease)

Etiology:
- Unknown
- Histopathologically, obliterative vasculitis of small and middle-sized arteries and veins
- Typical disease of heavy smokers

- Men are affected more often than women
- Genetic predisposition (HLA-A9 and HLA-B5)

General involvement:
- Due to lack of arterial blood supply:
  - Absence of pulsation, claudication
  - Ulceration of the finger tips and toes
  - Raynaud's syndrome
  - Thrombophlebitis (40%)

Ocular involvement:
- Vasculitis of the retinal vessels

Diagnosis:
- Clinical picture
- Laboratory tests: ESR normal
- Doppler sonography and angiography to confirm obstructions

Literature:
1. *McKusick VA, Harris WS, Ottesen OC, et al.:* Buerger's disease: a distinct clinical and pathogenic entity. JAMA 181: 5-122, 1962

3.68 Lymphomatoid granulomatosis

Etiology:
- Unknown
- Histopathologically, vascular infiltration with mature and atypical lymphocytes

General involvement:
- Similar to systemic symptoms in Wegener's granulomatosis with pulmonary, renal and central nervous system involvement
- Mortality 63%
- Frequent transition to malignant lymphoma

Ocular involvement:

- Diplopia
- Chorioretinitis
- Retinitis associated with infiltration of the vitreous
- Vasculitis of the venules and arterioles

Diagnosis:

- Clinical picture
- X-ray examination reveals diffuse pulmonary infiltration
- Biopsy confirms the diagnosis

Remarks:

Seemingly a rare disease.

Literature:

1. *Kinyoun LJ, Kalina RE, Klein ML:* Choroidal involvement in systemic necrotizing vasculitis. Arch Ophthalmol 105: 939-942, 1987
2. *Pearson ADJ, Craft AW, Howe JM:* Choroidal involvement in lymphomatoid granulomatosis. Br J Ophthalmol 75: 688-689, 1991
3. *Tse DT, Mandleboum S, Chuch DA, et al.:* Lymphomatoid granulomatosis with ocular involvement. Retina 5: 94-97, 1985

3.69 Frosted branch angiitis

Etiology:

- Unknown, possibly viral
- Young persons contract the disease (33 is the maximum age in the literature)

General involvement:

- Occasionally prodromal signs of a viral infection (e.g. fever)

Ocular involvement:

- Sudden onset
- Severe vascular sheathing of the veins; at times, and to a lesser degree, also of the arteries
- No vascular occlusions
- Central, extending into the periphery
- Severe visual impairment due to cells in the vitreous and occasionally also in the anterior chamber
- Unilateral or bilateral
- Spontaneous healing, possibly facilitated by corticosteroids
- Can leave scars
- Favorable prognosis

Diagnosis:

- Fluorescein angiography:
  - Late stage: leakage
- Electrophysiology: ERG shows diminished amplitudes

Literature:

1. *Kleiner RC, Kaplan HJ, Shakin JL, et al.:* Acute frosted retinal periphlebitis. Am J Ophthalmol 106: 27-34, 1988
2. *Sugin SL, Henderly DE, Friedman SM, et al.:* Unilateral frosted branch angiitis. Am J Ophthalmol 111: 682-685, 1991
3. *Watanabe Y, Takeda N, Adachi-Usami E:* A case of frosted branch angiitis. Br J Ophthalmol 71: 553-558, 1987

3.70 Eales' disease

Etiology:

- Unknown
- May be induced by immunologic mechanisms
- More common in men
- Age of onset usually less than 40

General involvement:

- Occasionally labyrinthine hearing loss and dysequilibrium

Ocular involvement:

- Obliterative vasculitis:
  - Venous vessels affected
  - Onset peripheral, progressing towards the posterior pole
  - Initial involvement of the optic nerve is rare (Differential diagnosis: central vein occlusion)
  - Very slight vitreal reaction
  - Vitreal hemorrhage
  - Tractional detachment
  - Occasionally spontaneous healing

Diagnosis:

- Fluorescein angiography:
  - Neovascularization
  - Areas of nonperfusion
  - Arteriovenous shunts

Literature:

1. *Rennie WA, Murphy RP, Anderson KC, et al.:* The evaluation of patients with Eales' disease. Retina: 3: 171-178, 1983
2. *Spitznas M, Meyer-Schwickerath G, Stephan B:* The clinical picture of Eales' disease. Graefe's Arch klin exp Ophthalmol 194: 73-85, 1975
3. *Wessing A, Lossagk H:* Beidseitige akute Periphlebitis unbekannter Genese. Ber dtsch ophthalmol Ges 71: 636-639, 1972

G) Postoperative uveitis/endophthalmitis and masquerade syndromes

3.71 Uveitis following cataract extraction

Etiology:

- Acute iridocyclitis (toxic-lens syndrome):
  - Supposedly caused by the chemical influence of the artificial lens
  - 2–4 days after implantation of an artificial lens
  - Possibly an acute form of chronic iridocyclitis
- Chronic iridocyclitis:
  - Reaction to intraoperatively transmitted infections
  - The most important pathogens appear to be:
    - Propionibacterium acnes
    - Staphylococcus epidermidis
    - Achromobacter
  - The incubation period varies widely (2 months to 2 years postoperatively)
  - Variability of the incubation period is attributable to:
    - Varying degrees of encapsulation
    - Differences in pathogenicity
    - Severe pathogenicity can lead to endophthalmitis
- Fulminant recurrence
  - Following cataract extraction in uveitis patients
  - Probably caused by insufficient suppression of the immune system, which responds vehemently to the surgical trauma
  - Appears also to depend on the type of uveitis (see vol. 2)
  - Onset soon after the operation
- Sterile anterior chamber inflammation:
  - Occurs to varying degrees after nearly every cataract extraction, probably independently of the extent of surgical trauma

General involvement:

- None, in contrast to endogenous endophthalmitis

Ocular involvement:

- Acute iridocyclitis (toxic-lens syndrome):
  - Severe pain
  - Marked visual impairment
  - Fibrinogenesis, synechiae, hypopyon
  - Vitreal reaction
  - Brief drop in IOP followed by a rise
  - Probably very rare today
- Chronic iridocyclitis
  - Chronic irritation of the anterior chamber
  - White deposits on the lens or haptic are typical
  - Occasionally hypopyon
  - Responsiveness to steroids is initially good, later poor
  - Transition to endophthalmitis or panophthalmitis is possible
  - No particular high-risk groups have been described to date
- Fulminant recurrence:
  - May result in barely controllable inflammation
  - Occasionally with fibrin exudation
  - Tendency to hypertonia followed by hypotonia (possibly phthisis bulbi)
  - Pain is rare

Diagnosis:

- History:
  - The onset of inflammation gives important clues for the differential diagnosis
- Clinical picture:
  - Slit-lamp examination may reveal typical white infiltrates in chronic iridocyclitis
- Laboratory tests:
  - Identification of possible pathogens

- Anterior chamber or, better, vitreal puncture specimen
- Inoculation of culture media, to be observed for at least 7 days
- Anaerobic cultures should also be used

Remarks:
New generations of intraocular lenses have led to the extinction of the classic 'toxic-lens syndrome' (which was caused by contamination of or deposits on the lens).

Literature:

1. *Foster CS, Fong LP, Singh G:* Cataract surgery and intraocular lens implantation in patients with uveitis. Ophthalmology 96: 281-288, 1989
2. *Manners RM, Canning CR:* Posterior lens capsule abscess due to Propionibacterium acnes and Staphylococcus epidermidis following extracapsular cataract extraction. Br J Ophthalmol 75: 710-712, 1991
3. *Michelson B, Friedlaender MH, Nozik RA:* Lens implant surgery in pars planitis. Ophthalmology 97: 1023-1026, 1990

3.72 Postoperative or exogenous endophthalmitis

Etiology:
- Endophthalmitis is exogenous in 90% of patients
- Contracted intraoperatively (49-75%) or by perforating injury (16-23%)
- Usually a continuous transition from anterior uveitis
- Transition depends on:
  - Pathogenicity of the causative agent
  - Predisposition: diabetes mellitus, lowered resistance
- Spectrum of bacterial pathogens:
  - Staphylococcus epidermidis (40-60%)
  - Staphylococcus aureus
  - Streptococcus sp.

- Propionibacterium acnes
- Proteus sp.
- Pseudomonas aeruginosa
- Achromobacter
- Hemophilus influenzae
- Serratia marcescens
- Spectrum of mycotic pathogens:
  - Fusarium, Aspergillus, Candida, Acremonium
- Postoperative:
  - Cataract extraction (90% of postoperative forms of endophthalmitis) (cf. Chapter 3.70)
  - Nd:YAG capsulotomies

General involvement:
- None

Ocular involvement:
- Iridocyclitis (following cataract extraction) or
- Primary endophthalmitis (following perforating injury)
- Painful
- Responsiveness to steroids is initially good, later poor
- Bacterial endophthalmitis:
  - Onset usually within the first postoperative week
  - Fulminant or chronic course
  - Prognosis: unfavorable
- Mycotic endophthalmitis:
  - Onset sometimes after months, but has also been reported within the first postoperative week
  - Tendency to chronicity
  - Micro-abscesses of the cornea, iris or vitreous
  - Unfavorable prognosis, even after correct diagnosis and therapy
  - Prognosis depends on:
    - Vision at first examination or diagnosis
    - Type of fungus: Acremonium and Fusarium have the worst prognosis

Diagnosis:

- History:
  - Complaint of pain
  - Previous surgery or trauma
- Clinical picture: Sometimes of no help in establishing a diagnosis
- Laboratory tests:
  - Identification of pathogens:
    - Anterior chamber or, preferably, vitreal puncture specimen with membrane filtration
    - Positive findings in 75% of eyes diagnosed clinically as bacterial endophthalmitis

Literature:

1. *Affeldt JC, Flynn HW, Forster RK, et al.:* Microbial endophthalmitis resulting from ocular trauma. Ophthalmology 94: 407–413, 1987
2. *Neuteboom GH, de Vries-Knoppert WA:* Endophthalmitis after Nd:YAG laser capsulotomy. Doc Ophthalmol 70: 175–178, 1988
3. *Puliafito CA:* Endophthalmitis: advances in diagnosis and therapy. Curr Op Infect Dis 3: 559–562, 1990

3.73 Post-traumatic uveitis

Etiology:

- Postcontusional
- Reactivation of herpes simplex virus from the ciliary ganglion seems possible
- During immunosuppression, e.g. in AIDS, reactivation of varicella zoster is also possible
- In many cases of uveitis, the connection with previous trauma is unclear and difficult to ascertain
- Since diverse autoimmune diseases can be induced by mechanical impact as in a trigger reaction, this might also be possible in uveitis

General involvement:

- None

Ocular involvement:

- Keratitis dendritica (HSV)
- Keratouveitis (HSV, VZV)
- Anterior uveitis

Diagnosis:

- Clinical picture and history:
  - In HSV reactivation: Time since trauma. Onset of keratitis/uveitis 2 to 5, possibly 7 days after trauma

Remarks:

Typical HSV keratitis and, in certain cases, uveitis are currently the only diagnoses accepted in expertises for medico-legal purposes.

Literature:

1. *Rosenbaum JT, Tammaro J, Robertson JE Jr:* Uveitis precipitated by nonpenetrating ocular trauma. Am J Ophthalmol 112: 392–395, 1991
2. *Sundmacher R:* Trauma und Herpes. Fortschr Ophthalmol 81: 409–415, 1984

3.74 Intraocular lymphoma

Etiology:

- Unknown
- Infiltration by B-lymphocytes, rarely T-lymphocytes
- 5-year survival in 20%

General involvement:

- CNS involvement in 25%, in which case:
- Weakness, headache, disorientation

- With unilateral ocular involvement the disease often affects the ipsilateral hemisphere of the brain

Ocular involvement:
- Initially unilateral; in 75-80% of cases the other eye becomes involved after a period ranging from several months to years
- More common in elderly patients, but also described in a 27-year-old
- Intermediate uveitis
  - Vitreous cells are larger than usual and become clumped
- Occasional hypopyon
- Tumor infiltration of the retina and choroid:
  - Whitish-yellow infiltrates
  - Very diverse clinical picture
  - Exudative, thickened areas are common
  - Exudative retinal detachment can occur
- Ocular symptoms can precede CNS involvement by 1 to 10 years

Diagnosis:
- Laboratory tests:
  - Diagnostic vitrectomy:
    - Reveals large pleomorphous cells with a narrow plasma border, interspersed mitoses, prominent nuclear membranes and invaginations
  - Puncture specimens of the anterior chamber usually yield no tumor cells
- Ultrasound diagnosis

Remarks:
An intraocular lymphoma should always be taken into consideration if a state of intraocular inflammation has resisted all treatment over months and/or has not led to a massive impairment of function. The term 'reticulum cell sarcoma' is inappropriate and should be avoided.

Literature:

1. *Char DH, Ljung BM, Miller T, Phillips T:* Primary intraocular lymphoma (ocular reticulum cell sarcoma). Diagnosis and management. Ophthalmology 95: 625-630, 1988
2. *Faulborn J, Daicker B, Bowald S:* Zur Klinik und Histopathologie des sogenannten Retikulumzellsarkoms des Auges. Klin Mbl Augenheilk 183: 120-121, 1983
3. *Kim EW, Zakov ZN, Albert DM, et al.:* Intraocular reticulum cell sarcoma: a case report and literature review. Graefe's Arch Klin Exp Ophthalmol 209: 167-178, 1979

3.75 Masquerade syndromes

Ischemic ophthalmopathy:

- Caused by insufficient arterial vascularization
- Usually associated with carotid stenosis
- Inflammation of the anterior chamber
- Rubeosis iridis
- Recurrent amaurosis fugax
- Diagnosis: Doppler sonography

Retinal detachment:

- Leads to cellular infiltration of the vitreous, possibly also of the anterior chamber
- Differentiation of a previous non-prominent retinal detachment from uveitis can be a problem, particularly in the case of intense vitreal irritation
- Bulbar hypotonia often occurs
- Diagnosis: ultrasound examination

Posterior vitreal detachment:

- Can on occasion lead to cellular vitreal infiltration
- Diagnosis: ultrasound examination

Vitreal hemorrhage:

- Sometimes indistinguishable from underlying uveitis
- Occasionally found in pars planitis and other forms of uveitis
- Exclusion of diabetes mellitus
- Diagnosis: ultrasound examination

Orbital pseudotumor:

- Benign, inflammatory orbital infiltration
- Cellular infiltration of the anterior chamber when the anterior orbit area is primarily affected
- Possibly associated with hypopyon
- Usually dull pains
- Absence of the typical mixed congestion at the limbus
- Usually exophthalmos
- Diagnosis: ultrasound examination, computed tomography

Choroidal melanoma:

- Inflammatory picture in 5-10%
- Can lead to an iridocyclitis-like picture
- Possibly vitreal hemorrhage
- Diagnosis: transillumination, ultrasound examination

Retinoblastoma:

- Growth is occasionally diffuse
- Inflammatory picture in 10-20%
- Requires exclusion in all intraocular inflammations leading to severe irritation where examination of the fundus yields insufficient information
- Invasion of the anterior chamber is possible, similar to hypopyon, with flaky, lime-white deposits
- Can present as panuveitis
- Diagnosis:
  - Ultrasound examination
  - Cytological examination of puncture specimen of the anterior chamber or vitreous can reveal cells with pale cytoplasm and prominent nucleoli

  - Laboratory tests:
    - Elevated lactate dehydrogenase activity in the aqueous humor

Intraocular metastases:
- The most common intraocular tumors
- Breast carcinoma and pulmonary carcinoma are the most common primary foci

Granuloma annulare:
- Develops as a yellow tumor between pars plana and equator
- Can lead to retinal detachment
- Diagnosis: ultrasound examination

Juvenile xanthogranuloma:
- Anterior chamber cells, possibly associated with pseudohypopyon or hemorrhage
- Diffuse infiltration of the iris and ciliary body
- Usually affects children, but not always

Hodgkin's disease:
- Granulomatous iritis:
  - Occasionally with hypopyon
- Retinopathy:
  - Cotton-wool spots
  - Periphlebitis
  - Exudative retinal detachment
  - Retinal hemorrhage
- It appears possible that many of the described ocular changes are attributable to secondary diseases, e.g. VZV retinitis

Leukemia:
- Gray, spotty leukemic retinal infiltrates
- Intraretinal and preretinal hemorrhage
- Vitreal hemorrhage

- Cellular vitreal infiltration
- Serous retinal detachment
- Papilledema
- Additional CNS symptoms are possible
- Diagnosis: puncture of the anterior chamber and vitreous, examination of the extracted cellular material

Paraneoplastic syndromes:

- Carcinoma-associated retinopathy
- In particular in parvicellular pulmonary carcinoma
- The tumor appears to produce an antigen similar to a retinal antigen, thus provoking production of autoantibodies
- Absence of vitreal infiltration
- Diagnosis: history, ERG sharply reduced

Radiation retinopathy:

- Follows, e.g. brachytherapy, application of radioactive plaques, helium ion or proton irradiation
- From appr. 3000 cGy upward, in case of additional chemotherapy even with 1200 cGy
- Onset appr. 7 months to several years after irradiation
- Possibly damage to vascular endothelium and pericytes of the retina
- Cotton-wool spots, intraretinal and vitreal hemorrhage, microaneurysms, retinal capillary telangiectasis, macular edema, vascular sheathing, neovascularization

Schwartz syndrome:

- 'Cells' in the aqueous with secondary glaucoma
- Associated with retinal detachment in patients with retinal holes
- Material in the anterior chamber consists mainly of photoreceptor components

Scleritis:

- Occasionally associated with cellular infiltration of the anterior chamber or vitreous body
- If associated with vasculitis, scleritis usually develops only after retinal or uveal involvement and can then be regarded as a more severe manifestation of vasculitis
- Diagnosis: sonography in posterior scleritis

Literature:

1. *Char DH, Schwartz A, Miller TR, Abele JS:* Ocular metastases from systemic melanoma. Am J Ophthalmol 90: 702-707, 1980
2. *Rosenthal AR:* Ocular manifestations of leukemia. Ophthalmology 90: 899-905, 1983
3. *Thirkill CE, Roth AM, Keltner JL:* Cancer-associated retinopathy. Arch Ophthalmol 105: 372-375, 1986
4. *Lopez PF, Sternberg P, Dabbs CK, et al.:* Bone marrow transplant retinopathy. Am J Ophthalmol 112: 635-646, 1991
5. *Fraser DJ, Font RL:* Ocular inflammation and hemorrhage as initial manifestations of uvea malignant melanoma: Incidence and prognosis. Arch Ophthalmol 97: 1311-1313, 1979

Abbreviations

Ab:	Antibody
ACE:	Angiotensin Converting Enzyme
AIDS:	Acquired Immune Deficiency Syndrome
ANA:	Antinuclear Antibody
ANCA:	Anti-Neutrophilic Cytoplasmic Antibody
AC:	Anterior Chamber
APMPPE:	Acute Posterior Multifocal Placoid Pigmentary Epitheliopathy
C:	Cornea
CMV:	Cytomegalovirus
CREST syndrome:	Syndrome including Calcinosis cutis, Raynaud's phenomenon, Esophageal motility disorder, Sclerodactyly and Telangiectasia
DD:	Differential Diagnosis
EBV:	Epstein-Barr Virus
ECM:	Erythema Chronicum Migrans
EOG:	Electrooculogram
ERG:	Electroretinogram
ESR:	Erythrocyte Sedimentation Rate
FTA-ABS test:	Fluorescent Treponemal Antibody Absorption test
HIV:	Human Immunodeficiency Virus
HLA:	Human Leukocyte Antigen
HSV:	Herpes Simplex Virus
IOL:	Intraocular Lens
MEWD syndrome:	Multiple Evanescent White-Dot Syndrome
PCR:	Polymerase Chain Reaction

PSS:	Progressive Systemic Sclerosis
RNA:	Ribonucleic Acid
RPE:	Retinal Pigment Epithelium
SLE:	Systemic Lupus Erythematosus
TBC:	Tuberculosis
TINU syndrome:	Tubulo-Interstitial Nephritis and Uveitis syndrome
V:	Vitreous
VDRL test:	Venereal Disease Research Laboratory test
VKH syndrome:	Vogt-Koyanagi-Harada syndrome
VZV:	Varicella zoster virus

Subject index